MW01614824

Breastfeeding Management for Physicians & Other Healthcare Providers

6th Edition

Anne Eglash MD, IBCLC, FABM
Kathy Leeper MD, IBCLC, FABM
Gail S. Hertz MD, IBCLC, FABM

The Little Green Book of Breastfeeding Management for Physicians & Other Healthcare Providers

Anne Eglash MD, IBCLC, FABM
Kathy Leeper MD, IBCLC, FABM
Gail S. Hertz MD, IBCLC, FABM

Published by The Milk Mob
PO Box 930445
Verona, WI 53593-0442

https://themikmob.org

6th Edition
Rev. 6.0 – March 2017
Copyright © 2017
ISBN: 978-0-9987789-0-7

Dedication

We dedicate this book to the generous families with whom we continue to learn the art and science of breastfeeding.

Special Thanks

Mitch Rosefelt for design and layout

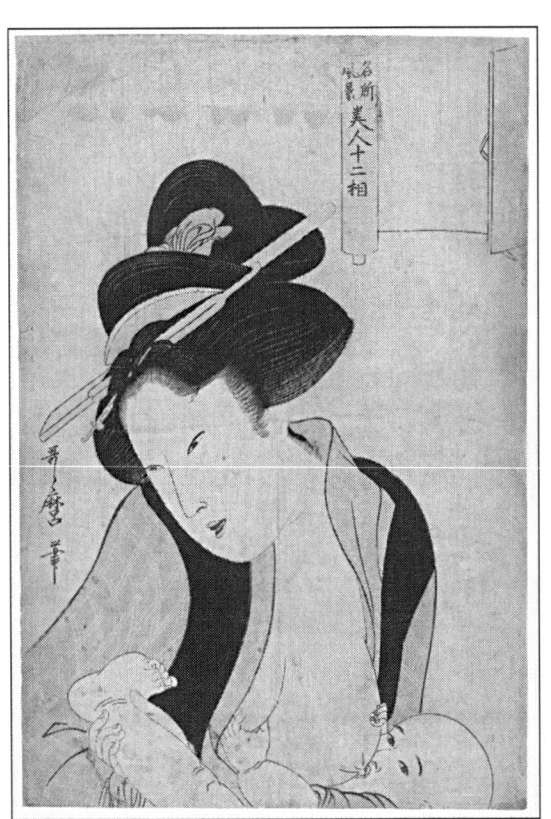

Table of Contents

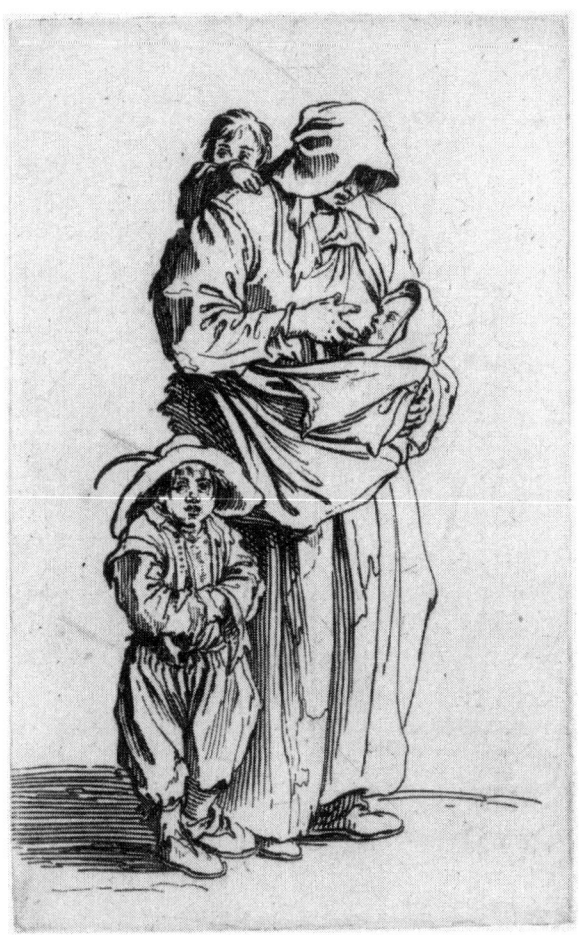

Bioactive Factors in Breastmilk

Breastmilk is a complex biological fluid containing over 200 'living', active components, many of which are known to complement the newborn's immature immune system. These bioactive factors provide nutrition, fight pathogens, reduce inflammation, promote the establishment of a healthy gut microbiome, and facilitate growth and maturity of the immune system. For example, breastmilk is very rich in IgA antibodies, which provide direct antimicrobial protection throughout the infant gut and other mucosal surfaces such as the nose, throat, and eustachian tubes. Breastmilk has a rich diversity of oligosaccharides, which are complex carbohydrates that promote the growth of healthy bacteria for the infant gut. In addition, oligosaccharides act as decoys of intestinal epithelium. Pathogens attach to oligosaccharides in the infant gut rather than attaching to epithelial cells. This strategy prevents invasion of pathogens, reducing the risk of diarrhea and respiratory infections. Lactoferrin, a dominant protein in breastmilk, is nutritional, antimicrobial, and has been found to enter infants' intestinal cells via lactoferrin receptors, acting as a transcription factor on the cell's DNA to synthesize immune proteins.

Human milk is a dynamic fluid that differs from mother to mother. Its composition changes from feeding to feeding and over the course of time from newborn to toddler. The unique qualities of mother's milk comprise the normal food for her infant, providing unparalleled protective and nutritive properties.

Why Is It Important to Breastfeed?

Two systems compensate for the immature immune system of the newborn: placental transfer of maternal antibodies and the transmission of many immunoprotective and immunomodulating factors through breastfeeding. While the effects of placental transfer wane by six months of age, the delivery of immune support and maturation from breastmilk is available to the child the entire time he is breastfed. The benefits appear to last even beyond the age of weaning.

The American Academy of Pediatrics, the American Academy of Family Physicians, and the American College of Obstetrics and Gynecology, all affirm that breastfeeding is protective of many diseases for the infant and mother. The health outcomes for infants and mothers ought to be measured using breastfeeding as the physiologic norm. The health risks for formula-fed infants compared to breastfeeding infants include an increased risk of diarrhea; 100% increased risk of otitis media; leukemia; 250% higher risk of hospitalization for a lower respiratory infection; 56% increased risk of Sudden Infant Death Syndrome; obesity; and type 1 and type 2 diabetes mellitus. A meta-analysis published in the Lancet January 2016 added an increased risk for dental malocclusion, and a higher risk of a lower IQ. For premature infants, rates of necrotizing enterocolitis (NEC) are higher in formula-fed infants.

For maternal outcomes, a history of lactation is associated with a reduced risk of type 2 diabetes, and women who do not breastfeed have a higher risk of breast and ovarian cancer. More than two years of lifetime lactation was found to reduce myocardial infarction risk in a large prospective cohort, and this association persisted after controlling for multiple lifestyle factors.

It has been estimated that if 90% of infants in the US were breastfed according to medical recommendations, 3,340 annual excess deaths would be prevented, 78% of which are maternal due to myocardial infarction (n = 986), breast cancer (n = 838), and diabetes (n = 473). Excess pediatric deaths total 721, mostly due to Sudden Infant Death Syndrome (n = 492) and necrotizing enterocolitis (n = 190). Medical costs total $3.0 billion, 79% of which are maternal. Costs of premature death total $14.2 billion.

In addition to the health benefits, breastmilk is always the right temperature, needs no mixing, is ready when infant is, and it's free. It is species-specific and changes in composition for the age of the child. Mother's milk supply will adjust to the infant's needs. Mom doesn't need to carry bottles, bags, and ice packs to go out. Families with breastfed children save money and create less waste for the environment.

How to Read the Literature

The volume of breastfeeding literature has grown exponentially in recent years. Conducting studies on the health effects of breastfeeding is challenging, in part because it is not ethical to randomize subjects to a non-breastfeeding group, due to the documented health risks associated with not breastfeeding. There can also be biases in research questions, or potential conflict of interests on the part of the investigators, particularly if there are ties to the pharmaceutical, formula, for-profit milk banking, or infant feeding industries. In evaluating a study, notice who sponsored the study and how the authors categorized breastfeeding groups.

There is a dose-response gradient demonstrating that the greater the proportion of breastmilk in the infant's diet, the greater the difference in health outcomes between infants who are breastfed as compared to infants not breastfed.

It is important that studies use the accepted standard definitions for breastfeeding. The exclusively breastfed infant receives only breastmilk at the breast – no formula, water, teas, or porridges. The exclusively breastmilk-fed infant may receive milk from a cup, bottle, or other vessel, as well as at the breast. A partially breastfed infant receives some other substance besides breastmilk – yet many studies categorize these infants as "breastfed." The ever breastfed infant may only have gone to breast one time in the hospital or perhaps stopped breastfeeding once at home.

Studies that do not distinguish between these groups or are vague in defining breastfeeding will have questionably valid results.

Special Conditions Necessitating Breastfeeding Caution

Infant health problems

- Infants with galactosemia type 1 are usually unable to breastfeed- other subtypes may be able to partially breastfeed
- Maple syrup urine disease
- Phenylketonuria- Phenylalanine in breastmilk is low, so women can partially breastfeed

Maternal Health Problems

- **HIV:** According to the World Health Organization Guidelines 2016, lactating mothers with HIV who stay on anti-retroviral medication, and who have undetected viral load may continue to breastfeed. Maternal treatment with anti-retroviral medications prevents transmission of HIV through breastmilk.

- **HTLV I and II** - Limited breastfeeding may be possible after discussing risks and benefits with the infant's healthcare provider.

- **Herpes simplex and herpes zoster (shingles)** If the lesions are directly on the nipple/areolar area, the mother needs to temporarily pump and discard her milk from the affected breast to avoid infant exposure to the infectious lesions. The infant may continue to nurse from the breast that is unaffected. Mother may continue to nurse on both breasts if sores are not on the nipple/areolar region, as long as the infant does not come into direct contact with the sores (e.g.

if sores are on arm and upper chest, mom should keep those covered).

- **Illicit Drugs** - Mothers abusing heroin, methamphetamines, cocaine and PCP should not breastfeed. Occasional, not daily, marijuana use is not a strict contraindication to breastfeeding, although this is controversial.
- **Certain Medications-** See the medication section. The vast majority of medications are compatible with breastfeeding.

Current Breastfeeding Recommendations

The American Academy of Family Physicians, the American College of Obstetrics/Gynecology, and the World Health Organization all recommend that infants exclusively breastfeed for 6 months. This means that no other foods, water, or formula should be offered to infants younger than 6 months. The American Academy of Pediatrics recommends exclusive breastfeeding for around 6 months. After 6 months breastfeeding should continue, with the introduction of appropriate complementary foods, through at least 1-2 years and beyond. Culturally, it is considered normal and acceptable for mothers to breastfeed their children until two years and beyond for the many nutritional, immunologic and developmental benefits. There is no evidence indicating an age at which breastfeeding should cease.

Anatomy/Physiology

The breast, or mammary gland, is the only organ not fully developed at birth. It undergoes four developmental stages: in utero, during the first two years of life, at puberty, and during pregnancy and lactation. During puberty, breast growth consists of ductwork, fat and connective tissue to support the ducts. The ultimate size of the breast is determined mainly by the amount of fatty tissue in the breast and is usually unrelated to milk production.

The nipple contains smooth muscle fibers and sensory nerve endings. Size and shape varies from woman to woman. Nipple pores are openings in the milk ducts on the face of the nipple and range from 1 to 18 in number. The areola is the darker pigmented area from which the nipple protrudes in the center. The areola will enlarge and darken over the course of pregnancy. Within the areola are the Montgomery glands or tubercles. They secrete a lubricating substance that both conditions and protects the nipple and areola from infection. Occasionally milk can be expressed from these glands.

During pregnancy the placental hormones direct the breasts to develop alveolar tissue, usually resulting in a significant increase in size or fullness in the breasts. Alveoli within the glandular tissue are lined with milk-making cells called lactocytes that respond to prolactin by drawing nutrients from the mother's blood in order to manufacture milk. Myoepithelial cells surround each alveolus and duct and contract in response to oxytocin, creating the 'let-down' or milk ejection reflex (MER). The force of these contractions propels milk through the milk ducts, which terminate at the nipple pores. The ducts and ductules form a complex network which is neither symmetrical nor radial in its pattern. (See Figure 1).

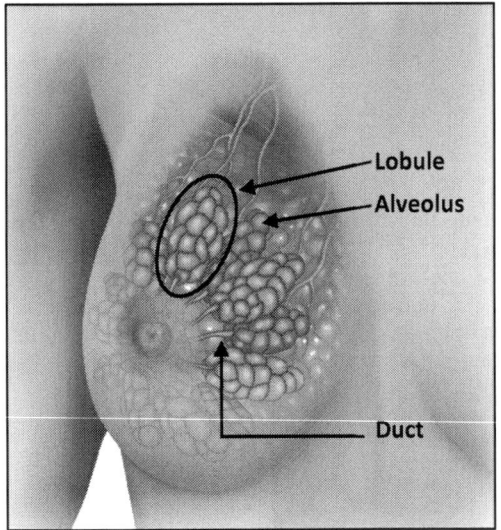

Fig 1.

In lactogenesis I, the breast responds to the circulating prolactin during pregnancy and manufactures early milk called colostrum, beginning at about 16 weeks gestation. Colostrum is thick, yellowish in color, rich in antibodies and beta carotene. Full milk production is inhibited by the placental hormones, particularly progesterone. Once the placenta is delivered and progesterone abruptly declines, lactogenesis II occurs, leading to increasing volumes of colostrum over the next 2-5 days. Women feel a sudden increase in breast fullness which is referred to as "the milk coming in". Breastmilk in the first few weeks postpartum is termed transitional milk, as it is higher in protein and yellow in color, as compared to white mature milk, which develops by day 14 postpartum. Mature milk's composition changes slightly based on the fullness of the breast and the overall daily volume produced. Mature milk of a mother with a term infant averages 20 kcal/oz (67 kcal/100 ml).

Prolactin and oxytocin are the two major hormones involved in lactation. Prolactin is high during pregnancy and peaks at the time of delivery. Baseline prolactin levels gradually fall over the first several months postpartum. Nipple stimulation causes a temporary doubling of the blood level. If a mother does not remove milk at all after delivery, her prolactin falls to pre-pregnancy levels within 2 weeks. The prolactin hormone is essential to lactation, and nipple stimulation is required to maintain elevated levels. However, baseline levels of prolactin do NOT directly correlate with milk production volume. Prolactin levels fluctuate, with higher levels overnight and in the morning, and lowest levels in the evening. This may be one major reason why mothers observe that they make more milk in the night.

Oxytocin, also called the "love hormone," is released not only when mom is nursing but also in response to other stimuli such as thinking about, hearing, seeing, smelling, or touching the infant. Oxytocin causes contraction of myoepithelial cells surrounding the milk ducts and alveoli, propelling milk out through the nipple. This is called the milk ejection reflex or "let-down". The release of oxytocin creates pleasant feelings of affection and calmness in the mother, supporting attachment to her infant and positive parenting behaviors. The calming effect of oxytocin decreases the mother's response to stress. This conditioned oxytocin release can be inhibited by stress, anxiety, pain, alcohol or opioids.

Counseling Families on Infant Feeding Decision and Prenatal Support

Research has shown that mothers are greatly influenced by what their healthcare providers do and do not say.

In 2016 The United States Preventative Services Task Force recommended that physicians provide interventions during pregnancy and postpartum to support breastfeeding.

One strategy to introduce a conversation about breastfeeding is to simply ask patients during early pregnancy 'How do you plan to feed your infant?' Most mothers have made a preliminary decision by early pregnancy whether they will breastfeed or not. After asking her plans for infant feeding, the conversation can segue into the reasons why she is choosing to breastfeed or not. Common barriers to breastfeeding include employment concerns, perceived inconvenience, lack of social support, embarrassment about breastfeeding in public, and a history of breastfeeding problems in the past.

If she is choosing to not breastfeed, this is an opportunity to dispel any myths or address perceived barriers to breastfeeding success. Women who decide to not breastfeed need informed consent regarding the maternal and infant health risks of not breastfeeding.

Although breastfeeding is 'natural', success requires health education for the mother, partner, and any involved family members before the infant is born. Prenatal breastfeeding education needs to include the risks of not breastfeeding, basic breastfeeding skills such as positioning, latch, infant feeding cues, frequency of feedings, and signs of adequate milk intake. Women should also learn how to manage common challenges such as engorgement and sore nipples.

Prenatal education may occur in a formal structured group (class) setting, 1:1 education by the prenatal provider, peer counseling, or other community organizations in the USA such as La Leche League or WIC (Special Supplemental Nutrition Program for Women, Infants and Children).

The University of North Carolina has excellent free resources for prenatal breastfeeding educational tools that can be used by health professionals and other breastfeeding supporters:

http://breastfeeding.sph.unc.edu/prenatal-breastfeeding-education-tools-and-recommendations-for-action-links/

It is never appropriate to give pregnant women samples of infant formula. Infant formula gift packs are only gifts to the formula companies that are being promoted. Formula gift packs give a message to the mother that she is not expected to be successful with breastfeeding. Appropriate prenatal gifts could include child safety-locks for the home, infant clothing, books, educational resources, or something special for the mother such as a gift certificate for a massage.

Prenatal Red Flags for Breastfeeding Problems

A few pre-existing conditions are associated with insufficient milk supply postpartum. These include a personal history of low milk supply in the past, a history of breast reduction surgery, breast irradiation, infertility, gestational diabetes, morbid obesity, and polycystic ovarian syndrome. Because not all women with these conditions have a low milk supply postpartum, close follow-up with the mother and infant postpartum to ensure appropriate weight gain is warranted. Other than the certainty that an irradiated breast will not produce milk, there is no way to predict whether a woman with these conditions will have difficulty with a low milk supply, and to what degree.

Breastfeeding Policies that impact public health

Baby Friendly Hospital Initiative

The Baby Friendly Hospital Initiative, was developed by the World Health Organization and UNICEF in 1991 as a means of increasing breastfeeding rates, in order to decrease infant mortality. Hospital policies in compliance with the "Ten Steps" of the Baby Friendly Hospital Initiative have been shown to increase breastfeeding initiation and duration, and maternal-infant bonding.
http://www.infantfriendlyusa.org/about-us/infant-friendly-hospital-initiative/the-ten-steps

The Ten Steps:

1. Have a written breastfeeding policy that is routinely communicated to all healthcare staff.

2. Train all healthcare staff in skills necessary to implement this policy.

3. Inform all pregnant women about the benefits and management of breastfeeding.

4. Help mothers initiate breastfeeding within one hour of birth.

5. Show mothers how to breastfeed and maintain lactation, even if they should be separated from their infants.

6. Give newborn infants no food or drink other than breastmilk, unless medically indicated.

7. Practice rooming-in, allowing mothers and infants to remain together 24 hours a day.

8. Encourage breastfeeding on demand.

9. Give no artificial teats or pacifiers (also called dummies or soothers) to breastfeeding infants.

10. Foster the establishment of breastfeeding support groups and refer mothers to them on discharge from the hospital or clinic.

International Code of Marketing of Breastmilk Substitutes (The Code)

The International Code of Marketing of Breastmilk Substitutes was adopted in 1981 by the World Health Assembly (WHA) as a means of preventing the formula industry from decreasing breastfeeding rates thru their marketing practices. The WHA recommended that all countries pass legislation to enforce this code of ethics regarding the sales and marketing of artificial baby milk. The United States has never enforced The Code. In countries where The Code is enforced, companies are prohibited from advertising to parents, offering free samples, and idealizing artificial feeding. The provision of free hospital discharge bags containing formula or coupons is one marketing strategy proven to undermine breastfeeding success. The bags are known to decrease the duration of breastfeeding, thus putting infants at higher risk for morbidity and mortality, in addition to increasing the risk of maternal illnesses among mothers who do not breastfeed. Many states have passed legislation banning the distribution of free formula gift bags. For more information, see https://banthebags.org/

The United States Joint Commission's Pregnancy and Related Conditions hospital core measure set was revised in 2010 to include Exclusive Breastmilk Feeding. This has served to motivate hospitals to improve breastfeeding support.

The Immediate Postpartum Period

The Golden Hour

The first hour after an infant is born is very important to ultimate breastfeeding success. A healthy, term infant should be placed "skin-to-skin" and chest-to-chest immediately after a vaginal or cesarean birth, as newborns have the instinctive ability to find their way to the nipple and self-attach within one hour. Sedating medications can have a negative effect on self-attachment, however every healthy infant should be placed skin-to-skin and given the opportunity to self-attach right after birth.

Skin-to-skin

On-going skin-to-skin contact (SSC) with the newborn beyond the golden hour can facilitate continued optimal latching and frequent feeding. SSC also decreases crying and stabilizes the infant's physiological functioning and metabolism, as evidenced by blood sugars on average 10mg/dL higher than if not SSC. For optimal safety, the newborn should wear just a diaper and be placed between mom's breasts with the legs flexed, the head slightly extended and turned to one side, and the body (not face) covered by a blanket. For the first hour or two, physical assessments and any necessary care can be done while the mom and infant are skin-to-skin.

As per the 2016 American Academy of Pediatrics Statement Entitled Safe Sleep and Skin-to-Skin Care in the Neonatal Period for Healthy Term Newborns "The main concerns regarding immediate postnatal SSC include sudden unexpected postnatal collapse (SUPC), which includes any condition resulting in temporary or permanent cessation of breathing or cardiorespiratory failure. Many, but not all, of these events are related to suffocation or entrapment." This statement suggests that because these events often occur in the first few hours of life, "it is prudent to consider staffing the delivery unit to permit continuous staff observation with frequent recording of neonatal vital signs." The mother and her support

people should also be educated on safe positioning while SSC.
LINK:
http://pediatrics.aappublications.org/content/early/2016/08/18/peds.2016-1889

Positioning and Latch

It is important for both mother and infant to be comfortably yet properly positioned for feedings. Excellent videos about latch and positioning are available from Global Health Media (www.globalhealthmedia.org/videos/) or The Milk Mob (www.themilkmob.org). It is best if mother is either laying back 45 degrees for "infant-led" latch, or sitting straight up, rather than bent forward, for "mother-led" latch. In any case, the infant should have the ear, shoulder and hip in alignment to allow for a deep latch and optimal oromotor coordination. Side-lying, with both mother and infant lying on their sides on a flat surface facing each other, is another option.

Once both are comfortable, either the infant self-attaches, or mother offers the breast using the asymmetric latch method, by pointing the nipple towards the nose or upper lip. (See figure 2).

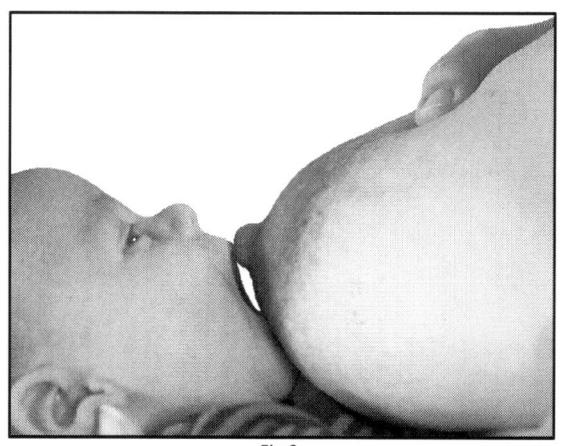
Fig 2.

This helps facilitate a deep, asymmetric latch, with the newborn latching beyond the nipple, and onto the breast tissue behind the areola. A deep latch, beyond the nipple, optimizes milk removal because the infant needs to compress and massage the breast tissue in order to remove milk. Latching onto the nipple alone leads to compression of the nipple between the tongue and palate, causing nipple trauma with open sores. In addition, such shallow latching is associated with poor milk removal, because the nipple does not have milk-producing glandular tissue, and the nipple becomes obstructed when the nipple ducts are compressed.

Rooming-In

Having mother and infant in the same room during their hospital stay is the best way for mom to learn and respond to her newborn's feeding cues. Crying is a late sign of hunger, and it is generally more difficult for the infant to organize and latch well when crying or agitated. Forced separation, even for vital sign checks and physician rounding, is not necessary since nearly all infant cares, labs, treatments, and exams can be done in the mother's room. This affords the primary care provider an opportunity to talk to and educate the parents during the exam, pointing out findings and reassuring the parents. Taking the infant to the nursery at night has not been shown to improve maternal quality or quantity of rest. Finally, separation makes frequent feedings less likely. Frequent milk removal is essential for optimal milk production and to minimize infant weight loss.

Feeding Frequency

Variations in breastfeeding rhythms occur between mothers and among cultures. Nursing patterns can vary from 8-20 feedings a day. A single feeding is often defined as the infant nursing from one or both breasts, with an interval of 1-3 hours from the start of one feeding to the start of the next feeding. Non-nutritive sucking is defined as a series of sucks with very few swallows. The sucks may appear in an irregular pattern, and are short. Little milk transfer occurs during this period. This suckling pattern often occurs at the beginning of a feeding, and stimulates the milk ejection reflex. Non-nutritive suckling also occurs at the end of a feeding when milk flow has slowed and the infant is relaxing or sleeping. Nutritive sucking is a slower, more rhythmical pattern with a wider mouth excursion. There are one or two sucks per swallow and milk is transferred. An audible swallow makes a quiet "cuh" sound.

Mother's colostrum volume at a single feeding matches the newborn's very limited stomach capacity. Colostrum has laxative properties and is easily digested, so the infant may want to nurse very frequently, such as every 1-3 hours, or 10-12 times in 24 hours. The frequency and effectiveness of milk removal is the most important driver of production throughout lactation: REMOVE IT OR LOSE IT. It is very important that healthy, term newborns are not "scheduled" to feed, as they do best if they eat very frequently while waiting for the transitional milk to "come in". It can be impossible to wake a infant in a very deep sleep when the clock says it is time to eat. A term healthy newborn will typically have one good feeding right after birth and then sleep for several hours on the day of birth. As long as mom and infant are in close proximity, ideally skin-to-skin, feedings should naturally resume when infant is ready. An infant who is having difficulty waking up to nurse at least 7-8 times in 24 hours by day 2 may need coaxing to wake up and nurse at least every 3 hours to maintain hydration and to maximally stimulate mother's breasts to establish a healthy milk supply.

Pacifiers

The routine use of pacifiers in the full-term newborn can interfere with the establishment of breastfeeding by interfering with frequent nipple stimulation and milk removal. It is recommended that pacifier use be delayed until about 3 weeks, when breastfeeding is well established.

Weight Loss

Always weigh infants completely naked and ideally on the same scale. It is normal for an infant to lose weight during the first few days after birth. The infant weight loss will level off around day three to four when mom's milk increases in volume. It is important to have a weight done on the day of hospital discharge, in order to determine the change in weight at the first outpatient visit. An infant who is feeding effectively should lose no more than seven to ten percent of birthweight. An infant who has lost more than 7% of birthweight during the hospital stay should be evaluated by a lactation specialist to assess feeding effectiveness.

Stools

The first stool should occur within the first 24 hours of life. This will be meconium—a thick, black, sticky substance. This stool gradually becomes looser and transitions to a brownish-green color, then finally yellow. The yellow stool may be "seedy" and is the consistency of pancake batter. New parents often voice concern that the typical breastfed stool has the appearance of diarrhea. During the first 2-3 days of life, there may be anywhere from a few to several meconium stools each day. By day 4, infants typically have approximately four "credit card size" yellow seedy stools per day. This change occurs as mom's milk increases in volume ("comes in") and is a good indication of how well breastfeeding is going. Moms who have breastfed a previous child tend to see the milk increase by day 2-3, as compared to a mom with her first child, for whom the milk supply typically increases by day 3-5.

Problems during the Postpartum Hospitalization

Jaundice

All newborns should be screened for hyperbilirubinemia, whether the screening is clinical, transcutaneous, or blood sampling.

Breastfeeding infants tend to have higher physiologic total serum bilirubin levels compared to infants who are formula feeding. Studies indicate that 30-40% of breastfed infants have total serum bilirubin levels >5mg/dl at 3-4 weeks of age. There are 2 main reasons why breastfed infants have higher bilirubin levels:

1. Breastfeeding infants have a higher risk of excessive weight loss and lack of sufficient calories during the first week postpartum. This can be due to a delay in the milk coming in, infant feeding problems such as latch or sleepiness with lack of sufficient milk transfer, or maternal-infant separation leading to infrequent feeding. Lack of sufficient calories leads to higher levels of unconjugated bilirubin, at least partially due to increased intestinal reabsorption of bilirubin. Increasing calories with associated increased stooling helps to resolve the hyperbilirubinemia.

2. Breastmilk jaundice is a condition that starts as an exaggerated early physiologic jaundice in the first week. These infants continue with fairly high

bilirubin levels for the next several weeks. The bilirubin level will gradually drift down over the course of 8-12 weeks. Suspected mechanisms include underlying Gilbert's syndrome, with underactivity of the UGT1A1 enzyme responsible for glucuronidation of bilirubin. Breastmilk is also known to suppress the UGT1A1 enzyme activity. Breastmilk jaundice has been observed to rapidly resolve by interrupting breastfeeding for 24 hours and feeding the infant cow's milk-based formula. Formula is known to induce UGT1A1 activity. However, because the level of bilirubin in cases of breastmilk jaundice tends to be harmless, there is rarely a medical indication to interrupt breastfeeding.

Kernicterus is the most concerning outcome of hyperbilirubinemia. Infants at highest risk for kernicterus are late preterm infants who have insufficient breastfeeding skills, with excessive weight loss. Late preterm infants have immature livers and weak blood brain barriers, allowing serum bilirubin to move more easily into extravascular spaces of the brain. Late premature infants who are not feeding well, especially if they have an ABO incompatibility or bruising, are at very significant risk for excessively high and dangerous bilirubin levels. Many hospitals have special feeding protocols for late preterm infants to help maintain proper hydration and assist mother with breastfeeding plans for this population. (See Late Preterm Pg. 38)

The Academy of Breastfeeding Medicine's protocol on management of hyperbilirubinemia in

breastfeeding infants over 35 weeks gestation can be found at:
http://www.bfmed.org/Resources/Protocols.aspx

Hypoglycemia

Routine blood glucose screening of healthy newborns is NOT indicated. Healthy, term, low-risk newborns do not develop clinically significant hypoglycemia due to limited duration or frequency of breastfeeding. Evidence indicates that routine blood sugar testing for healthy infants can lead to negative consequences for breastfeeding.

There are several newborn risk factors for which blood glucose screening is recommended, such as small for gestational age, large for gestational age, infants of diabetic mothers, prematurity, among others. The Academy of Breastfeeding Medicine protocol on management of hypoglycemia for the breastfeeding infant can be found at:

http://www.bfmed.org/Resources/Protocols.aspx

If an asymptomatic newborn is screened due to a risk factor and found to have a serum glucose low enough to require IV glucose administration, frequent breastfeeding should be encouraged.

Delay in Lactation

'Delay in lactation' is a term used to describe a situation where the newborn is still losing weight and there is no sign of milk "coming in". The mother perceives a lack of breast enlargement and/or fullness by the end of day 3 for a multip and day 5 for a primip. A delay in lactation results in the need to supplement the infant because of excessive weight loss. A thorough evaluation by a lactation specialist is recommended in these situations. The mother is usually instructed to begin expressing milk after breastfeeding, either by hand or using a breast pump. The infant will need supplementation with whatever expressed breastmilk is available, in addition to donor milk or formula. A firm feeding plan and close follow-up are needed to support the dyad.

If the mother is able to express sufficient milk after nursing, this is not a delay in lactation but rather a situation where the infant is not transferring milk well. Infants who are not transferring well also need an evaluation by a lactation specialist.

Indications for Supplementation

A supplement is any milk given to an infant in addition to direct feeding at mom's breast. The first choice for supplementation is mom's own expressed breastmilk, followed by pasteurized donor breastmilk. Hypoallergenic (extensively hydrolyzed) formulas are a third choice. Supplementation should never be water, sugar water, other animals' milk or any other liquid.

Supplements should be given only when medically necessary. Infants who receive a supplement after breastfeeding might not breastfeed as often. If the breasts are not emptied when the infant is supplemented, mother's milk supply may decrease because the infant is not draining the breast as often. Because milk production is a supply-demand phenomenon, a decrease in milk removal will send a message to the breasts to produce less milk. The goal of supplementation is to meet the infant's needs while the supply at the breast is maintained, or increased if necessary.

Some common medical indications for supplementation are:

- Hypoglycemia that is not controlled by frequent breastfeeding, see section on hypoglycemia
- Jaundice, when the infant has evidence of insufficient calorie intake
- Physical or laboratory signs of dehydration
- Maternal illness requiring maternal infant separation
- Contraindications to breastfeeding (see section on Special Conditions Necessitating Breastfeeding Caution p. 13)

The Academy of Breastfeeding Medicine's 'Clinical Protocol #3 on Hospital Guidelines for the Use of Supplementary Feedings in the Healthy Term Breastfed Neonate' can be found at http://www.bfmed.org/Resources/Protocols.aspx

Options for Supplementation

It is difficult to predict which newborn will have difficulty transitioning back to the breast after using a bottle. Paced bottle feeding using a slower-flowing nipple may be helpful to prevent bottle preference.

Infant-paced bottle feeding is intended to keep the infant from the "drink or drown" situation, caused by milk pouring into their mouth. The infant should be sitting upright, and caregivers are taught to read infant's cues and pace the feeding to give infant control of his own intake and prevent overfeeding (see figure 3).

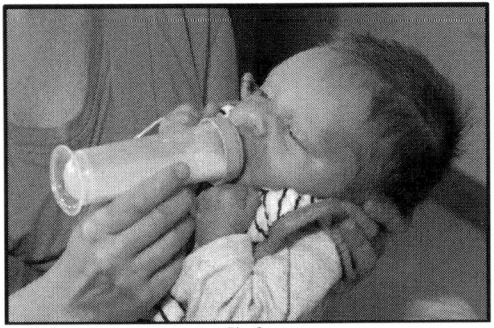
Fig 3.

The Infant Who Will Not Latch

Sometimes infants do not latch-on to the breast right after birth, and other times they will have a few good nursing sessions the first day and then not latch-on again before leaving the hospital. There are several reasons why this might happen. The following are fairly common:

- The infant is sleepy and/or premature, and does not sense the breast tissue in his mouth.

- For whatever reason(s), the infant received bottles right after birth.

- The milk supply is low in the hospital, and the infant is frustrated and too impatient to sustain nursing.

- The infant has a tongue-tie or other physical or motor issue, such as torticollis or pain.

- The breast is very difficult to grasp either for maternal or infant reasons.

If a newborn is unable or unwilling to latch, mother can hand express colostrum into a spoon and offer it to infant every 1-3 hours until infant latches or her milk "comes in". Hand expression is ideal for the small volumes of sticky, thick colostrum. Once her breasts are increasing milk production, she may find that using a breast pump is more effective, especially combined with manual expression.

If the infant is not latching by discharge, evaluation by a lactation specialist is important to sort out the underlying reason. The family will need a feeding plan at the time of discharge, along with coordination of care for follow-up as outpatients.

Sore Nipples

Nipples may be somewhat sensitive during the first few days postpartum, but significant pain is not normal. Nipple cracks, scabs, and bleeding are also not considered normal. If a mother has sore nipples in the first few days of breastfeeding, the most likely cause is a latch problem. (See latch and positioning p. 24) If the nipples are intact, mother can apply some expressed breastmilk or lanolin after nursing, to keep the nipples supple. If there are open wounds, an antibiotic ointment and a nonstick covering are important to allow for moist wound healing, and to prevent the open wounds from sticking to the bra or breast pad.

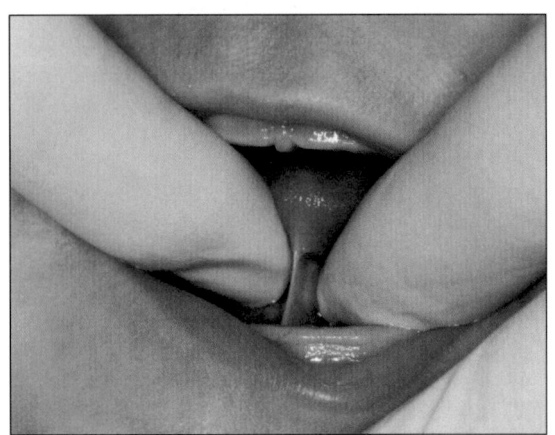
Fig 4. Tongue-Tie Pre-treatment

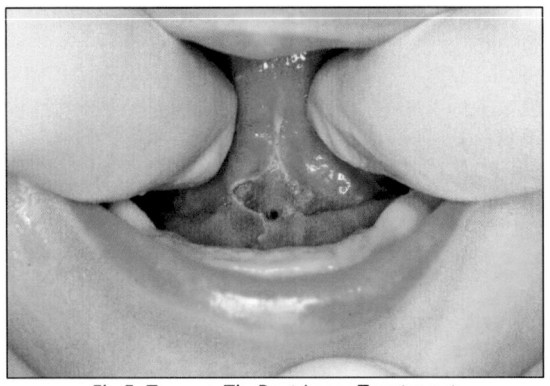
Fig 5. Tongue-Tie Post Laser Treatment
Photos courtesy Kristen Berning DDS

Tongue-Tie

Lingual frenula (see figs 4 & 5), also known as tongue-ties or ankyloglossia, can restrict tongue movement, making it difficult for the infant to latch deeply, and/or maintain a deep latch during feeding. The consequences of shallow latching are nipple pain, nipple trauma, and insufficient milk transfer, resulting in inadequate infant weight gain and a drop in milk supply.

Tongue-ties are often described as anterior and posterior:

Anterior tongue-tie

These are visually apparent as either a thin or thick tissue (frenulum) attaching the underside of the tongue to the floor of the mouth, limiting tongue movement.

Posterior tongue-tie

These are often not visually apparent, but can be felt by sweeping a finger under the tongue. A 'speed bump' or thick band may be felt at the base of the tongue. Oftentimes, these do not need to be clipped. Signs of breastfeeding problems related to a posterior tongue-tie include lack of sufficient milk transfer despite a healthy milk supply, or persistent pain with feeding. Lactation specialists are able to identify subtle suck and swallow behaviors indicating that a posterior tongue-tie may be causing a feeding problem. Before having a posterior tongue-tie clipped, the infant should be evaluated by a lactation specialist who has the skills to discern whether the feeding problem is related to the posterior tongue-tie.

It is not uncommon to identify a newborn with an anterior lingual frenulum while still on the postpartum unit. If the mother and infant are not having feeding problems such as latch problems, milk transfer difficulties, or nipple pain, it is not necessary to clip the frenulum before discharge. The mother should be informed that her infant has a lingual frenulum and be educated about possible breastfeeding problems including nipple pain and problems with infant weight gain or maternal milk supply. Not all infants with an anterior tongue-tie need to have a frenotomy. Occasionally an anterior lingual frenulum needs to be clipped before hospital discharge, particularly in cases of significant nipple pain despite optimal positioning and latch strategies. It is highly unlikely that a posterior tongue-tie needs clipping before discharge. Breastfeeding dyads who are having problems should be monitored by a lactation specialist over time, before determining that the breastfeeding problems are related to a posterior tongue-tie as opposed to other possible problems. (for more information on tongue-tie, see page 37)

Late Preterm

Infants born between 34-37 weeks gestation are at higher risk for breastfeeding difficulties as compared to term infants. Late preterm infants have a higher risk for hypothermia, hypoglycemia, and physiologic hyperbilirubinemia. In addition, they tend to be more sleepy at the breast and run the risk of insufficient milk transfer at the breast. It is reasonable to routinely supplement these infants in the early postpartum, until they demonstrate the ability to support themselves at the breast without supplementation. Late preterms ought to room-in with their mothers and feed ad lib. However, because they tend to be sleepier, they should be awakened to feed at least every 3 hours until mother's milk has increased, and the infants are nursing well on their own without supplementation.

Mothers should be encouraged to express their colostrum or early milk after nursing, and offer expressed breastmilk to the infant after each feeding. If she is not able to express her own milk, approximately 5-10ml of either donor milk or formula should be offered to the late preterm after nursing on day 1, followed by 10-30ml offered after feedings on day 2 and possibly day 3, depending on mother's milk supply, infant weight, and infant feeding skills. More details on breastfeeding the late preterm can be found in The Academy of Breastfeeding Medicine's protocol #10 entitled 'Breastfeeding the Late Preterm and Early Term Infants, Second Revision 2016' http://www.bfmed.org/Resources/Protocols.aspx

Prematurity/NICU

For newborns who are admitted to the neonatal intensive care unit (NICU), for prematurity or illness, breastfeeding is more challenging. The maternal-infant separation is a barrier to establishing mother's milk supply, and the infants often don't have the opportunity for early feedings at the breast. Mother should be instructed to express milk by hand AND with a quality breast pump within 2 hours after birth, and regularly at least every 3 hours with no more than a 5-hour break at night. A typical pump session lasts 10-15 minutes. Mothers should have a consultation with a lactation specialist regarding proper use of her breast pump, including proper shield size, ideal pressures, duration of pumping, and addition of massage and manual expression. The addition of manual expression to pumping has been shown to increase milk volume and fat in the milk. Pumping at the infant's bedside and covering the collection bottles with a blanket while pumping might yield higher milk volumes.

It is optimal to establish an abundant milk supply during the first seven to ten days, which is approximately 750-1000 ml/day. The single most important factor for mothers who will be breastfeeding a preterm infant at home is maintaining a milk supply that exceeds the infant's requirements at discharge.

Although this is a time-intensive routine, it empowers the mom at a time when parents may feel at a loss of how else to help their infant(s).

Skin-to-skin is of great benefit for the mother's mental health, her milk supply, and for infant's cardiorespiratory and neuro-sensory regulation.

The First Week After Hospital Discharge

The infant and mother need to be followed closely during the first week to monitor for excess weight loss, and to ensure that the mother is comfortable and gaining confidence. The first week postpartum is a common time for mothers to stop breastfeeding due to a delay in the milk coming in, excessive pain, excessive infant weight loss, or latch difficulties. With close follow-up, encouragement, education, and appropriate guidance on the management of breastfeeding problems, families are more likely to continue breastfeeding.

When to follow up after hospital discharge

Families are typically advised to see their pediatric health care providers within 24-48 hours after hospital discharge. Infants who are having feeding problems, jaundice, infrequent stooling, or moms with sore nipples should be seen within 24 hours after discharge.

Infants who are nursing well at the time of discharge, voiding and stooling appropriately, with a mother who feels that her milk supply is increasing may wait 48 hours to be seen.

For infants who have had a longer hospital stay, breastfeeding may be well established by hospital discharge, with mother's milk in and the infant already gaining weight. In these cases, the infant may be seen in 3-5 days after discharge.

First office follow-up visit

The first office visit postpartum often requires extra time to allow for breastfeeding questions, counseling about infant feeding patterns, cues and signs of feeding adequacy, and to troubleshoot issues such as sore nipples and engorgement.

History

Before asking questions, say something positive when walking into the exam room, such as 'you look so well rested' or 'your baby looks marvelous, what wonderful color!'. If the labor and delivery information is not known, ask details of the hospital events. Ask about frequency and duration of breastfeeding, the number of voids and stools, whether the stools are looking yellow and seedy. Ask about breast fullness, sore nipples, and whether she is having trouble with engorgement. Is the infant waking on their own to feed, satisfied after nursing and does the infant rest comfortably between feedings?

Exam

Exam details pertinent to breastfeeding include infant weight, jaundice, evidence for torticollis, nasal congestion, or tongue-tie, and general infant tone, hydration and wakefulness. On feeding exam, check for infant swallows and maternal comfort with breastfeeding.

<u>Reassuring findings</u>

Signs of breastfeeding adequacy - yellow seedy stools should be present once mother feels that her breasts are full, and the diapers should always be wet at that point. Stooling after each feeding in the first few weeks is considered normal. Mother notices that her breasts feel fuller before feeding, softer after feeding, and she notices swallows at the breast. Although frequent yellow seedy stools and many wet diapers are reassuring, weight gain is the only absolute proof of adequate infant intake.

Weight - weight loss should reach its nadir at 8-10% on day 2-4, then stabilize and rise as the milk is 'in'. Once mother's breasts feel full, an approximate 1 oz a day weight gain is very reassuring. If the infant's weight on day 3 is lower than at hospital discharge, see the infant back every 1-2 days until appropriate weight gain is established.

Topics of discussion during the first week

<u>Support at home</u>

Mothers and their partners need support during the first few weeks after birth. Most breastfeeding mothers need to nurse her newborn every 1.5-2.5 hours, so must rest between feedings and take care of their personal needs. Encourage families to accept help offered by others, such as caring for the other children, housekeeping, meal preparation, shopping, and running errands.

Vitamin supplements for mother and infant

Mothers are encouraged to eat 2-3 servings of seafood a week to boost the DHA (docosohexanoic acid) in her breastmilk, based on a 2014 Food and Drug Administration Cost-Benefit Analysis which included the risk of environmental contaminants. DHA plays a role in infant brain tissue development and adequate supplementation can boost infant IQ by approximately 3 points. All infants require vitamin D starting from birth. Because very few mothers have adequate vitamin D in their breastmilk, all breastfeeding infants are recommended to have 400 units of vitamin D supplementation. Infants born prematurely require iron supplementation. Term infants should not require iron supplementation, as long as complementary foods offered at 6 months are iron-rich. Delaying cord-clamping after birth for at least 1 minute or until the cord ceases pulsation allows for a normal physiologic blood transfusion to the infant at birth, decreasing the risk of iron deficiency in the first year.

Infant feeding schedule

A typical breastfeeding newborn nurses every 1.5-3 hours during the first 3-4 weeks. Infants often have times of very frequent feedings, or 'cluster feedings', characterized by nursing every hour during times of increased wakefulness, such as upon awakening in the morning, and in the evening. Breastfeeding may take 30-45 minutes for each feeding, depending on infant sleepiness and maternal milk supply. By 1-2 months of age, feedings may become shorter as the infant is less sleepy and more efficient. Mothers with a high supply and a fast let-down may find that feedings are considerably shorter. By 2-3 months of age, infants are often nursing every 2-3 hours during the day and night. By 4 months, it is normal for some infants to take 4-hour breaks between feedings.

Variations in milk supply

Mother's prolactin level is highest after she goes to sleep at night, and lowest in the evening, after being awake all day. Most mothers find that their milk supply is highest overnight and in the morning, and is the lowest in the evening.

Changes in stooling

 Once mother's milk has significantly increased by 3-5 days postpartum, infant stools become yellow, seedy, and appear watery. In the first few weeks, the stools may occur after each feeding. By 1 month postpartum, the infant's gastro-colic reflex calms down, and stooling will become less frequent, often 1-4 times a day. Some infants, particularly by 4 months of age, only have stools once a week, and occasionally less often. If interval weight gain is fine and the infant is comfortable and appears healthy, this is considered normal.

When to start pumping

 Nursing mothers often ask when to begin pumping to store breastmilk for work or other anticipated times of maternal-infant separation. Mothers should be encouraged to not pump for the first 3 weeks, unless they need to pump in lieu of nursing. Just nursing in the first 3 weeks allows the breasts to regulate to the nutritional needs of the infant. After 3 weeks, it would be reasonable to express right after the first nursing session in the morning, when the supply is highest. Limiting extra milk expression to no more than 2-4 ounces a day will help to decrease the risk of creating an over-supply of milk.

Night time feedings

It is normal for infants to wake up to nurse in the middle of the night. Infants vary greatly as to when they begin sleeping for longer stretches overnight. There is no evidence that it is safe to train infants to not awaken overnight, nor is there evidence that mothers should stop nursing at night to train their infants to sleep longer. Mothers who do not nurse or pump in the middle of the night run the risk of a drop in prolactin level, resulting in return of early menses, which often leads to an overall drop in milk supply. In addition, excessive fullness overnight can lead to a drop in supply due to local control factors in the breast tissue. For mothers whose babies naturally sleep all night at an early age, limiting the nursing or pumping breaks to 5-6 hours until 4 months and 7 hours after 4 months will help to prevent a drop in milk supply.

Common Breastfeeding Problems During the First Week

The infant who feeds "too often"

Breastfed infants tend to eat more frequently than formula-fed infants, and this can surprise parents. In the early days, 10-12 feedings a day (or more) is completely normal. Once the milk "comes in" at day 3-5, feedings often spread out somewhat, to every 1-

3 hours, or 8-12 times a day. It is normal for young infants to have times during the day when they cluster-feed, meaning that they feed every hour for 2-3 feedings in a row. This tends to happen when they are quite awake, such as in the morning or in the evening.

Infants who continue to feed every hour around the clock ought to be further evaluated. A weight should be checked and plotted on a growth curve, to be sure that they are transferring sufficient milk.

The most common reasons for excessive feeding frequency include:

- **Poor milk removal-** this would be identified by performing a pre and post-feed weight on a digital scale sensitive to 2 grams. If the infant takes a volume that only allows satiation for an hour, and the mother can express significantly more milk than what the infant took, then the infant didn't transfer milk well. This is often due to infant sleepiness at the breast, but can also be due to infant feeding problems such as gastroesophageal reflux, tongue-tie, or other health issues. A lactation specialist should be involved in evaluating this situation.

- **Maternal low milk supply**- Even if the infant is gaining adequately, the supply may be marginal, such that the infant needs to feed very often to gain sufficiently. The low supply can be from several causes, see the section on low milk supply p. 62. A subset of mothers with a low supply have a small amount of glandular tissue, meaning that they make small amounts of milk at one time. The infant has to feed often to obtain sufficient milk.

Parents may desire a plan to resolve such frequent feedings. If the infant is not removing sufficient milk, the mother will need to express milk after feeding and supplement the infant, while a lactation specialist determines the underlying problem and solution. If the mother's milk supply is low, the infant will need supplementation with donor milk or formula, as the lactation specialist determines how to help the mother increase her supply.

Slow Weight Gain

Once mom's milk supply is 'in', expected infant weight gain in the first 3 months is 20-30 grams a day. The infant's weights should be plotted on a World Health Organization growth curve to ensure proper interval growth. Healthy breastfeeding infants often reach birthweight before 2 weeks. Infants who are not gaining appropriately need evaluation by a lactation specialist to determine if the problem is lack of milk transfer at the breast, maternal low milk supply, or an infant health problem.

The sleepy infant

Many infants are sleepy in the first several weeks of life. This is especially true for premature or late preterm infants. The sleepiness can be most evident when the infant is nursing. Sleepy behavior at the breast is often coined 'living on the let-down', meaning that the infant will sleep at the breast until the milk ejection occurs. The sleepy infant will awaken sufficiently to swallow milk from the letdown, but won't continue to nurse effectively to continue milk transfer. This is the most common reason why a nursing newborn does not gain weight despite mother having an adequate supply. An initial approach is to teach parents strategies to keep the infant awake at the breast by stripping off clothing, tickling the feet and back, and teaching the mother to use breast compression to improve milk transfer.

Jaundice

See P. 29

Engorgement

This is interstitial swelling, or edema in tissues that surround the glands and ducts. This tends to be most severe in first-time mothers, and represents a fluid shift to the breasts early postpartum in order to begin the process of ramping up milk production. Engorgement can be uncomfortable and at times severe. It often leads to difficulty latching the infant onto the breast because the infant may not be able to compress the swollen, firm areola. Sore, cracked nipples are a common consequence of engorgement, due to shallow latching. Unrelieved engorgement may lead to a loss of milk supply due to involution of the milk-producing cells.

Every mother should receive anticipatory guidance on how to manage engorgement before she leaves the hospital. Education should include:

- How to manually express milk to soften the areola
- The use of ice or cold compresses while lying on her back to alleviate the swelling
- The importance of frequent nursing to prevent severe engorgement
- Reverse pressure softening as a technique of applying pressure on the areolar tissue circumferentially around the base of the nipple, to reduce areolar edema, allowing protrusion of the nipple, and enabling a deep infant latch
https://www.youtube.com/watch?v=2_RD9HNrOJ8
- Breast massage between and before nursing to help diminish swelling. An excellent resource for teaching breast massage is at http://bfmedneo.com/our-services/breast-massage/

Sore Nipples

Sore nipples are extremely common during the first few weeks postpartum. This is due to a variety of factors associated with lack of deep latching. Infant problems such as torticollis, tight jaw muscles, sleepy behavior at the breast, tongue-tie, and maternal problems such as eczema, very large nipples, inverted, or very flat nipples also contribute to sore nipples during the first few weeks.

The most important early interventions include optimizing the infant's position and latch in order to promote a deep atraumatic latch. The dyad may need to be seen by a lactation specialist for this. If skin is intact, some mothers find an emollient soothing, such as purified lanolin, when applied after nursing. If the mother has open nipple wounds, the principles of moist wound healing and preventing the wound from sticking to a surface will help to promote healing. (See Nipple Wounds Pg. 52) As long as the latch is no longer traumatic, her nipples will usually heal in a few days despite continued breastfeeding.

Depending on the degree of pain, mothers who need a break from nursing should be instructed to pump instead of breastfeeding. Pumping can also be traumatic, so it is important that she receive guidance on proper pump selection, shield size, and pump usage.

General Breastfeeding Medicine Topics

Acute Nipple/Breast Pain

Yeast Overgrowth

Yeast naturally lives on the surface of nipples, in balance with the bacterial microbiome. Several factors can affect this balance, such as antibiotics given for Group B strep or C-section. Symptoms are usually bilateral, and the regions of the nipple/areola complex taken in orally by the infant are typically bright red. The pain is described as "hot" or "burning". Yeast can be treated with a topical antifungal such as 1% clotrimazole cream twice a day, nystatin ointment 4 times a day or 1 % gentian violet applied once, repeating again in 3 days if symptoms persist. Oral fluconazole can also be used, 200mg once a day for 7-10 days. If the infant has visible oral thrush, the infant should also be treated with an anti-fungal medication.

Nipple Vasospasm

This is characterized by intermittent nipple pain, often described as "burning" or "stabbing" and shooting into the breast. It is typically associated with pale or purplish nipples, but color change is not always visible. Vasospasm can occur randomly, but most often with abrupt change in temperature, such as right after nursing, stepping out of a shower, or during pumping. Some mothers with vasospasm have a history of Raynaud's syndrome of the fingers and toes. Treatment involves keeping the nipples warm, applying dry heat over the bra or clothes right after nursing, and avoiding any nipple trauma. Calcium channel blockers such as nifedipine and verapamil have been used when the conservative measures are not sufficient.

Nipple Wounds

Occasionally open nipple lesions will continue after latch is corrected and engorgement resolves. If nipple sores persist, moist wound healing using non-stick pads and an antibiotic ointment such as mupirocin or bacitracin will help heal the nipples. It is important that the wounds not stick to the bra or breast pad, since this will lead to recurrent trauma to the nipples every time the bra flap is removed to nurse or pump.

The antibiotic ointment does not need to be taken off before the next nursing. If the nipple sores are not healing and intermittently oozing, consider a wound culture to rule out bacterial infection from staphylococcus aureus or other pathogens such as group A beta hemolytic streptococcus. It would also be reasonable to treat mother with an oral anti-staph antibiotic such as cephalexin, dicloxacillin, clindamycin or TMP sulfa.

Ongoing latch difficulties can perpetuate nipple trauma. Common causes of ongoing latch problems include infant tongue-tie, and infant oromotor dysfunction due to problems such as torticollis, tight or weak facial muscles. See the section on Infant tongue-tie (Pg. 37). Referring to a lactation specialist will help diagnose the possibility of other infant oromotor problems.

After teeth have erupted, the infant may cause wounds with their teeth, either from biting or the top teeth passively rubbing against mother's skin while feeding. Biting tends to occur at the end of a feeding, so mother can be encouraged to remove the infant a bit sooner than usual. Holding the infant very close also discourages pulling away to bite. If the top teeth are rubbing, rotating positions can be helpful.

Nipple Blebs

Nipple blebs are tiny white lesions at the tips of the nipples. There is controversy over the underlying etiology of these blebs, and there has been very little research done regarding the etiology or treatment of blebs. They have often been observed to occur in conjunction with deep plugs. They also might represent dissection of milk thru the walls of a nipple duct, creating lesions of subcutaneous trapped, inspissated milk. If the blebs are not painful, and there is not a plugged area in the breast, no treatment is needed. They will often resolve on their own. Occasionally un-roofing a bleb can be helpful to alleviate swelling and pain associated with the bleb, or relieve an associated plugged area in the breast. If unroofed, antibiotic ointment is recommended on the area regularly after nursing until the area heals, to decrease the risk of breast infection. The infant may continue to nurse regularly on the breast. If there is no sign of infection, another option for treatment is to apply a very small amount of medium strength topical steroid to the bleb, such as 0.1% triamcinolone ointment 3-4 times a day for 7-10 days.

Nipple Dermatitis

Dermatitis of the nipples can occur due to irritation from any substance coming into contact with the nipple, such as nipple cream or breast pads. It can also represent an allergic reaction, such as a penicillin-allergic mother who develops intense nipple redness, itching and swelling after coming into contact with amoxicillin given to her infant orally right before nursing. Women with a history of skin conditions such as eczema or psoriasis are at significant risk of having these same conditions affecting the nipples. Treatment involves identifying the underlying reason for the nipple dermatitis, with avoidance of any identified irritant or trigger. Repeated moisturization of the nipples after nursing is helpful using petroleum jelly or an oil such as coconut or olive oil. A medium strength steroid such as a 0.1% triamcinolone ointment is often necessary. The steroid should be applied sparingly after nursing. Once the dermatitis is under control, mother should be encouraged to gradually wean from the steroid ointment use. These substances do not need to be taken off before nursing.

Plugged Ducts

Plugged ducts are common occurrences during breastfeeding. Symptoms of a plugged duct include discomfort and engorgement in a section of the breast that is unable to drain due to a plug in the milk duct. The nipple and breast are often painful during nursing because traction on the duct causes pain. Risk factors for plugged ducts include high milk supply, irregular breast drainage due to a change in schedule such as working or infant sleep cycle changes, external compression such as tight clothing, and a nipple bleb. On exam, the breast may appear full in one area. Overlying redness or red streaking is not expected with an uncomplicated plugged duct, and would suggest a secondary mastitis.

Treatment is frequent nursing and/or pumping, breast massage, warm compresses, rest, and plenty of fluids. If the plugged region has not resolved by 2-3 days, an ultrasound is reasonable to further evaluate the lesion, in order to rule out an abscess, galactocele, or solid mass. Women should be warned about signs of mastitis. For some women with recurrent plugged ducts, lecithin capsules, 1200mg 4 times a day with weaning to the lowest effective dose has been helpful to decrease recurrences.

Acute Mastitis

Mastitis is defined as inflammation of the breast, and may or may not indicate an infection. Mastitis is most likely to develop during the first 2-3 months postpartum. Other risk factors for mastitis include over-supply, irregular feeding schedule, and persistent nipple sores. Women with mastitis often complain of flu-like symptoms such as body aches, headache, dizziness, nausea, fatigue, fever and chills. Mastitis is often preceded by a plugged duct.

During the early phase of mastitis, the breast may have a mildly pink area that is warm and tender. Over a few days, that pink area may progress to a deep, more expansive redness.

Treatment includes rest, analgesics such as acetaminophen or ibuprofen for pain and fever, warm compresses, massage and frequent nursing and/or pumping. If there is a high index of suspicion for infection (due to open wounds on nipple, lymphangitis, or toxic appearance of the mother) or symptoms do not improve after 12 hours of conservative management, then antibiotic treatment is warranted and should cover staphylococcus aureus, the most common bacterial cause of mastitis. Other pathogens causing mastitis include group B strep, staph epidermitis, enterobacter, E coli, and group A Beta-hemolytic strep, among others. Initial considerations for antibiotics may include dicloxacillin, cephalexin or another cephalosporin, amoxicillin-clavulanate, clindamycin, or TMP/Sulfa. Typical duration of antibiotic treatment is 10-14 days. Severe mastitis with high fever, signs of sepsis, and/or significant swelling and induration may necessitate hospitalization for parenteral antibiotics. A breastmilk culture is indicated if a woman is having recurrent mastitis, or her mastitis is not responding to appropriate antibiotic therapy. For further management guidelines, see The Academy of Breastfeeding Medicine protocol on mastitis.

http://www.bfmed.org/Resources/Protocols.aspx

<u>Abscesses</u>

Breast abscesses are walled-off regions of infection within the breast tissue, filled with purulent material. Usually an abscess occurs during the course of mastitis, and the mother presents with a firm mass in the breast with overlying redness. Occasionally a preceding mastitis was not apparent to the mother before presenting with a mass, and the mass is found on ultrasound to be an abscess. Treatment includes drainage of the abscess, ideally via percutaneous drainage using ultrasound guidance. The material removed needs to be sent for culture and sensitivity, and antibiotic treatment is warranted, usually for at least 10-14 days, or until redness and abscess fluid have resolved. After the initial percutaneous drainage, follow up ultrasounds and drainages should continue every 2-3 days until no more fluid is seen. Another option is placement of a catheter and drain by an interventional radiologist. Occasionally abscesses have too many septations to reasonably drain percutaneously, and need open incision and drainage. Breastfeeding women need to maintain continued drainage of the breast by nursing or pumping. If the milk is quite bloody and purulent, she may opt to express the milk and dump it temporarily, but in most cases the abscess will heal while the mother continues to breastfeed on that side.

Chronic Nipple/Breast Pain

Women may report several days or weeks of having deep dull aching breast pain or sharp shooting pains in the breasts, with or without breast tenderness. The symptoms may also include nipple pain and nipple sensitivity, painful milk ejection, and recurrent plugs. These women lack breast redness or other signs of acute mastitis.

Sorting out the underlying etiology of deep breast pain can be difficult, and referral to a lactation specialist is indicated.

The Academy of Breastfeeding Medicine's protocol entitled 'Persistent Pain with Breastfeeding' is helpful;
http://www.bfmed.org/Resources/Protocols.aspx

Several etiologies can be considered:

Oversupply

Some women generate more milk than the infant needs, and they suffer from heavy, uncomfortably full breasts. The breast pain in these situations is usually worse when the breasts are full. Bringing down the milk supply often alleviates the discomfort. See section on Hyperlactation (Pg. 68).

Vasospasm – See Pg. 52

Dysbiosis

The published literature regarding dysbiosis is largely within the bovine and goat literature, since it plays a major role in the quality of milk brought to market. It is thought to be an overgrowth of staphylococcus epidermitis, which is the commensal organism most commonly isolated in breastmilk cultures. A dysbiosis might also represent a change in the behavior of the staph epidermitis, with development of biofilm. Women may complain of intermittent deep breast aching and nipple pain with latching and between nursing. Some women have a history of recurrent plugged ducts, with a resulting decrease in milk supply. A history of acute mastitis is also common. The physical exam tends to appear normal, expect for breast tenderness on palpation. Occasionally the nipples have small yellowish scabs at the tips. A breastmilk culture and antibiotic treatment based on culture results is recommended. Antibiotic treatment may need to be extended 4-6 weeks, as long as steady improvement is occurring.

Yeast

Common symptoms of a candida infection of the nipples include burning nipple discomfort, nipple sensitivity, and sharp shooting into the breasts, which is referred pain from the nipples. It is unproven whether these women have yeast infections in their milk ducts deep within the breast. It is reasonable to consider treatment for superficial yeast overgrowth if a woman's nipples have a thrush- like appearance with red shiny skin, especially if satellite lesions are present. A KOH of a skin scraping from the nipple/areolar region can be helpful to make the diagnosis (see Yeast Overgrowth Pg. 51).

Imaging the Lactating Breast

A breast mass that is present for more than 3 days has a lower risk of being a simple plugged duct, and requires further evaluation with an ultrasound, and possibly a mammogram, depending on the protocol and skills of the imaging department.

Galactoceles

These are retention cysts filled with milk, thought to occur when a milk duct is obstructed. These are not typically tender on physical exam, and have no overlying redness or swelling. A galactocele can be left alone, and may not resolve until weaning.

Abscesses (see Pg. 57)

Solid breast masses

Breast masses require biopsy, just as they do for non-lactating mothers. Although there is a theoretical concern for a milk fistula following a biopsy, in reality these are very uncommon. Milk may flow from a biopsy site for a few days or weeks, but will gradually resolve.

Breast Surgery and Radiation

Women with a history of excisional biopsy rarely have problems breastfeeding. Breast augmentation usually does not impact breastfeeding other than an increased risk of engorgement if implants are very large. However, some women who have undergone breast augmentation have a history of insufficient glandular tissue. If the mother has a history of one or both breasts appearing significantly underdeveloped before surgery, she is at greatly increased risk of low milk supply.

Breast reduction surgery is much more likely to have a negative impact on milk supply because it generally involves removal of a large amount of breast tissue. These moms can usually breastfeed, but many will not bring in a full supply. Infants need to be closely monitored for milk intake and weight gain, and for this reason, nursing mothers with a history of breast reduction should receive care and guidance by a lactation specialist. Supplementation at the breast can help maintain the breastfeeding relationship and optimize production. A good online resource for breastfeeding mothers with a history of breast reduction is www.bfar.org.

Women with a history of radiation to one breast for cancer are not expected to produce any milk from the irradiated breast. Women who undergo radiation for other conditions such as Hodgkin's disease have much less radiation exposure to their breasts. These women should be watched carefully for adequate milk production, but are at lower risk for insufficient lactation.

Low Milk Supply

Perceived Low Milk Supply

There are many reasons why mothers PERCEIVE they are not making enough milk, when in fact they are. Breastfeeding is a confidence game. If a mother interprets infant feeding behavior or breast changes as a loss of milk supply she may decide to supplement the infant with formula, leading to a decrease in production due to less frequent feedings at the breast. Changes in feeding routines that mothers may interpret as low supply include:

- Feeding more frequently than expected
- Infants with a high suck need
- Constant infant fussiness
- Infant rejection of the breast
- Decline in breast fullness after 2-4 months postpartum
- Decrease in infant stooling
- Bottle preference

Mothers should be encouraged to see a provider or lactation specialist to help determine if these changes are due to low supply or something else. An infant weight is crucial to sort this out. Therefore, this is not an evaluation that can be done over the telephone.

Real Low Milk Supply

There are also many reasons why a mother has a truly low milk supply. It helps to divide causes of low milk production into problems originating prenatally, intrapartum, and postpartum.

Prenatal Causes of Low Milk Supply

The most likely prenatal cause of low supply is insufficient breast development, called "Insufficient Glandular Tissue" (IGT) or "breast hypoplasia". There are a variety of hormonal or anatomic problems associated with this phenomenon, all of which are not completely understood.

- **Hormonal**- breast development during pregnancy is under the influence of placental hormones that stimulate new glandular tissue formation. Hormonal problems such as polycystic ovarian syndrome, obesity, pre-eclampsia and diabetes are associated with insufficient glandular development during pregnancy. Current theories include high androgens and/or insulin resistance associated with these conditions.

- **History of breast procedures**- Women with a history of radiation to one breast, such as in cases of breast cancer, will not make milk from the irradiated breast. Breast reduction is also strongly associated with insufficient milk production. Breast augmentation tends to have little effect on milk production. (see section on Breast surgery and Radiation, Pg. 61)

- **Anatomic**- Some women have limited potential to make sufficient glandular tissue, for unknown reasons. These women may notice breast growth during pregnancy, but often have characteristic findings, such as wide spacing between breasts, a lack of 'rounding' of the breast, or tubular shaping of the breasts (See Fig 5). Women with very asymmetric breasts often find that the much smaller breast makes much less milk.

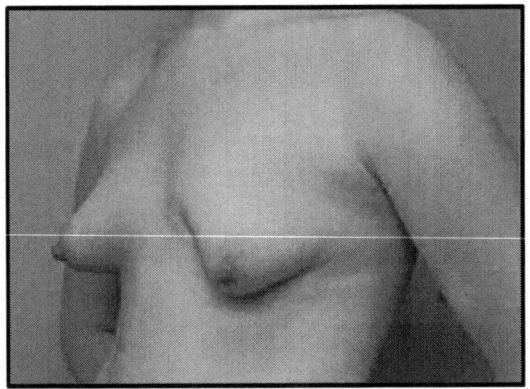

Fig 5.

Intrapartum Causes of Low Milk Supply

Some mothers have normal breast growth during pregnancy and no prenatal risk factors for low milk supply. Uncommonly, some mothers notice that the milk never 'comes in'. Reasons for this include:

- **Retained placental fragments**- Because the drop in progesterone after placental delivery is the hormonal trigger for making milk, retained placental fragments that continue to secrete progesterone can be associated with lack of lactogenesis II.

- **Pituitary trauma**- This is commonly known as Sheehan's syndrome, an infarct of the pituitary usually caused by extreme hypotension, which stops the release of prolactin and oxytocin, halting lactation.

- **Theca Lutein cyst**- These are ovarian cysts that secrete testosterone. Testosterone is a strong inhibitor of lactation.

- **Medications**- Some medications given postpartum can markedly impact milk production, including decongestants, high dose steroids, and progesterone given for contraception immediately postpartum.

If there is truly NO milk production, then an evaluation including serum cortisol, prolactin, testosterone, thyroid function testing, HCG, and possibly an ultrasound looking for retained fragments is indicated.

Postpartum Causes of Low Milk Supply

By far the most common scenario is that the milk does "come in" fine, but is not removed adequately, resulting in a low supply. REMOVING MILK FROM THE BREAST IS THE MOST POTENT STIMULATOR OF PRODUCTION. Lack of milk removal results in a build-up of the feedback inhibitor of lactation (FIL), which is a substance that communicates with the lactocytes to decrease milk production.

- Infrequent removal – this is often due to a sleepy newborn, scheduled feedings, limiting feedings due to sore nipples, supplementation, pacifier use, or not pumping often enough, such as at work

- Inadequate removal – often due to a shallow latch, tongue-tie, nipple shield, nipples too large for infant, exclusive pumping, cleft palate, recessed chin

- Maternal medications can also suppress production (See Maternal Medications Pg. 90)

When low milk supply is identified, mother should be referred to a lactation specialist, and thorough/frequent milk removal should be started immediately. Usually this would mean using breast compressions while breastfeeding, and pumping both breasts afterwards with a double-electric pump to remove as much milk as possible. Young infants often fall asleep when flow slows, and older infants become impatient and remove themselves too soon, leaving milk in the breast. This "triple feeding" (nursing, pumping and supplementing infant) is time- consuming and stressful. Some mothers will choose to pump and bottle feed when alone with the infant, and nurse the infant when someone else is home to help feed the infant while she pumps.

Galactogogues

Galactogogues are substances that increase milk production, and can be in the form of prescription medications, herbs, or foods. Complete and frequent milk removal is always the primary method for increasing milk supply. Galactogogues will not increase the milk supply if complete and frequent milk removal is not occurring.

The most common prescription galactogogues include metoclopramide and domperidone, both of which are manufactured for GI purposes, such as nausea, gastroesophageal reflux, and gastroparesis.

Metoclopramide is known to increase prolactin levels by inhibiting dopamine, and has been shown in some studies to as much as double the milk supply. It is not approved by the US Food and Drug Administration (FDA) for use as a galactogogue. Because metoclopramide crosses through the blood-brain barrier, central nervous system side effects are common, such as fatigue, dizziness, tremors, anxiety and depression. The risks of neurologic side effects increase with prolonged use, so if metoclopramide is used, the mother needs close monitoring, and duration should be limited to just a few weeks.

Domperidone also increases prolactin levels by inhibiting dopamine, and is as effective as metoclopramide in increasing the milk supply. It is much less likely to cross the blood brain barrier, so that neurologic side effects are uncommon. Domperidone is known to prolong the QT interval, so women at risk for arrhythmias or prolonged QT due to underlying heart disease or taking other medications should not take this. Domperidone is not manufactured in the United States, thus is not FDA-approved. The FDA considers it illegal to prescribe domperidone in the US. Domperidone is widely used in many other countries.

Many mothers turn to foods and herbs to increase the supply. There is limited information on their safety and effectiveness. Common substances believed to increase milk supply include fenugreek, alfalfa, ginger, caraway, fennel, blessed thistle, torbangun, moringa leaf, goats rue, and shatavari. Resources for further information on foods and herbs as galactogogues include:

- The Lactmed database of Toxnet, from the National Library of Medicine

- www.mother-food.com

- Academy of Breastfeeding Medicine Protocol entitled 'Use of Galactogogues in Initiating or Augmenting the Rate of Maternal Milk Secretion' http://www.bfmed.org/Resources/Protocols.aspx

- Natural Medicines Database www.naturaldatabase.com

Hyperlactation (Excess Milk)

It is possible for a mother to produce volumes of milk in excess of her infant's needs. A common cause is pumping after nursing, creating excessive demand for milk production. Some mothers do not excessively stimulate breastmilk production, and it is not well understood why their breasts don't down-regulate to match their milk production with the infant's demands.

Common infant symptoms include coughing and choking while nursing, especially with the first milk ejection, excessive weight gain, gas, frequent green explosive, watery stools, and/ or breast refusal.

Common maternal symptoms include breast fullness, frequent plugged ducts or recurrent mastitis, and sore nipples due to infant pinching to slow the flow.

Referring to a lactation specialist is a best strategy for management, as this process often must be individualized. Nursing in a "laid-back" position, with infant "on top", can help the infant handle the fast flow. Mom should also gradually decrease and ultimately stop any pumping in excess of infant's needs. If it is clear mom has an oversupply and a large storage capacity (>4oz per breast) she can try "block feeding", keeping infant on one breast for 3 hours at a time. This means that all feedings during that block of time, such as from noon to 3 pm, come from one breast. The mother then switches all feedings to the other breast from 3-6 pm, etc. If the side not nursed from becomes uncomfortably full, just a small amount of milk should be expressed for comfort. After 36-48 hours, the milk supply should down-regulate on both sides. At any time that the infant is no longer satisfied with just one breast, she should return to nursing her infant on both sides each feeding. This would signify that her oversupply has improved.

Occasionally a mother will not respond to leaving milk in the breasts. Pseudoephedrine has been shown to decrease milk production and prolactin levels. Single 30-60mg doses, repeated daily just as needed until the desired effect is seen, can be recommended. *Estrogen-containing contraceptives* can also be used, and it is advised to stop them when/if the supply has decreased in 5-7 days. Sage extract or sage tea is also very effective at decreasing the milk supply. It is used in a similar fashion to pseudoephedrine, 1 dose just as needed, usually not more than once a day.

Birth Control

Breastfeeding women who are exclusively breastfeeding during the first 6 months have lower fertility because of the Lactation Amenorrhea Method (LAM), which prevents ovulation. A woman who is fully or nearly fully nursing (no more than 1-2 supplementary feedings each week), is amenorrheic, and is under 6 months postpartum meets the criteria for LAM, and has an approximately 2% risk of pregnancy without birth control.

Contraceptive options that do not have an impact on lactation include barrier methods, such as condoms, diaphragms, and spermicides, and the copper IUD. Any hormonal methods can impact the milk supply.

The onset of milk production postpartum relies on the declining levels of placental hormones, primarily progesterone. Any progesterone, testosterone, or estrogen hormones given before breastfeeding is well established, usually at approximately 6 weeks postpartum, increases the risk of insufficient milk supply. Current recommendations from the Center for Disease Control and The World Health Organization differ on timing for the safe introduction of progesterone-only birth control and the combined estrogen-progesterone birth control products.

Unfortunately, the overall evidence is poor regarding the effect of hormonal contraception on the milk supply. Because estrogen and progesterone can block the prolactin receptors in the breast, there is a risk of lower milk supply with introduction of hormonal contraceptive methods even beyond 6 weeks postpartum. Evidence shows that estrogen is more likely to drop the milk supply than progesterone-only methods. Breastfeeding women need information to weigh the benefits of pregnancy protection with the risk of lower milk supply.

Many lactation specialists notice much less impact on milk supply with the progesterone IUD and the progesterone-only birth control pill when introduced at 6 weeks or later postpartum, in comparison with long acting progesterones. Placement of the progesterone IUD during the first few hours postpartum has not been well studied, and safety in terms of its effect on lactation has not been proven. The few studies done so far indicate that immediate postpartum placement of the progesterone IUD can be associated with insufficient milk supply.

Estrogen therapy is often quite effective to reduce milk supply at any time during lactation.

For more complete information on contraception during lactation, please see the Academy of Breastfeeding Medicine protocol entitled 'Contraception During Lactation' http://www.bfmed.org/Resources/Protocols.aspx

Maternal Illness

Surgery

A breastfeeding mother who needs surgery may continue to breastfeed. She may need coordination of care before, during and after surgery to help properly manage her lactation status, in order to prevent engorgement, plugs, infection, and loss of milk supply. If the surgery is elective, it is ideal for the primary care physician or surgeon to contact the hospital lactation specialist pre-operatively. The lactation consultant can assist with milk expression in the pre-op and post-op units, and during long surgeries. Anesthesia in breastmilk clears at the same rate as anesthesia in the brain, so once the mother is awake and alert after surgery, she can breastfeed her infant. It is ideal to allow the infant to room in with the mother post-operatively. She will most likely need a support person to stay with her to help manage the infant's needs.

Infectious Diseases

There are very few infectious diseases that preclude breastfeeding. If a mother has active tuberculosis, she needs to be isolated from her infant to avoid transmission thru respiratory secretions, but can provide expressed breastmilk. Mothers with HTLV type 1 or 2 are advised to not breastfeed. The World Health Organization's 2016 guidelines on HIV and breastfeeding suggest that mothers on anti-retrovirals who have no detectable viral load can breastfeed their infants. The Center for Disease control recommends separating a mother from her newborn if she is infected with influenza around the time of birth, until she is on anti-viral medication for 48 hours. She can continue to provide expressed breastmilk. Other illnesses such as hepatitis B and C are not contraindications to breastfeeding. Mothers with other infectious illnesses, such as gastroenteritis and mononucleosis, are encouraged to continue nursing. The IgA antibodies generated in response to an acute illness are transmitted to the infant via breastmilk, reducing the severity of illness for the infant. In addition, the other anti-infective and anti-inflammatory factors in breastmilk help reduce infant symptoms in the face of an acute infectious illness. The US Center for Disease Control's information on diseases and breastfeeding can be found at: https://www.cdc.gov/breastfeeding/disease/

Psychiatric Illnesses

Postpartum mood disorders are quite common. Women with a history of psychiatric illnesses such as depression prior to pregnancy are at high risk of recurrent mental illness postpartum. Maternal psychiatric illnesses such as psychosis, bipolar disorder, major depression and anxiety are sometimes seen as precluding breastfeeding because of the fear of exposing the infant to psychiatric medications. Research shows that most psychiatric medications are safe during breastfeeding due to low levels of transmission into breastmilk.

Stress and worry associated with breastfeeding problems can exacerbate depression and anxiety, but advising a depressed or anxious mother to stop breastfeeding has not been shown to improve depression, and may worsen depression.

Breastfeeding mothers with psychiatric disorders need support for their breastfeeding problems. They would also benefit from help regarding infant feeding at night, to improve their sleep quality and duration. This may involve having a helper bring the infant to the mother to nurse at night, with the helper caring for all of the other infant's needs overnight so that the mother can get back to sleep.

The Academy of Breastfeeding Medicine has a helpful clinical protocol entitle 'Use of Antidepressants in Nursing Mothers' http://www.bfmed.org/Resources/Protocols.aspx

Autoimmune Diseases

Mothers with autoimmune diseases such as Crohn's disease and rheumatoid arthritis are usually able to find disease-modifying agents that are compatible with breastfeeding. The National Library of Medicine's free Lactmed database, https://toxnet.nlm.nih.gov/newtoxnet/lactmed.htm, is an excellent source of information on medications in mothers milk. This database can be shared with breastfeeding mothers and medical specialists, such as rheumatologists, to decide on best medication options during breastfeeding.

New Onset Cancer

Occasionally a new mother develops cancer during pregnancy or postpartum. Breastfeeding mothers who require chemotherapy usually need to wean, since most, but not all, chemotherapy agents are contraindicated during breastfeeding. In addition, the mother needs her energy and nutritional resources for her own healing. Many mothers with cancer worry about their infants' health risks with artificial feeding, and may inquire about donor milk. Please see our section on donor human milk, Pg. 101.

Maternal Nutritional Challenges

Mothers who have risk factors for insufficient nutrients, such as veganism, short gut syndrome, and gastric bypass, should be assessed for repletion of vitamins, minerals and other nutrients. If the maternal levels are within normal limits, the breastfeeding infant will not need additional nutrient fortification, other than vitamin D (unless maternal vitamin D levels are moderately high, such as greater than 50ng/ml) and possibly iron.

Infant-Specific Breastfeeding topics

Infant Thrush

Infants with thrush are found to have white patches of yeast overgrowth on the buccal and/or lip mucosal surfaces, tongue, and throat. A white tongue by itself with no mucosal lesions is not typically thrush. Mothers often notice that the infant latch becomes more shallow as a response to oral discomfort. Treatment of oral thrush can include oral nystatin 4 times a day for 10-14 days, 1/2% gentian violet used sparingly once every 3 days, or oral fluconazole for 7-10 days. If the mother has no symptoms of nipple discomfort, she does not require treatment.

Infant Fussiness

Differentiating between infant fussiness and colic can be controversial, particularly because we don't have a clear etiology of colic. It is reasonable to assume that colic is normal for young infants from approximately 3 weeks to 3 months of age. Colic is often thought of as fussiness that occurs in a pattern, around the same time of each day, usually in the evening, and lasting for 3-4 hours, such as from 5 pm to 9 pm. During times of colic, babies are often hard to soothe, and they will often look to nurse more often. At all other times of the day, the infant is predictably pleasant and content.

Fussiness that occurs 24 hours a day is likely different than colic, and may represent another health problem such as intestinal upset, heartburn, ear pain, or some other sort of discomfort. Occasionally the maternal diet may play a role in chronic intestinal upset of a nursing infant. Removing dairy from mother's diet is a reasonable step in determining if a reaction to breastmilk is the cause of infant fussiness.

Infant Allergy and Sensitivity to Breastmilk

The food proteins from a mother's diet are found in breastmilk, and occasionally infants develop sensitivities and allergies to these food proteins. These reactions can present in several ways, such as eczema, reflux, or very infrequent stools accompanied by pain, or blood-streaked mucousy stools (proctocolitis).

Symptoms often appear between 3 and 6 weeks of age, but proctocolitis may present as late as 2-4 months of age. Food protein elimination from the maternal diet is recommended, starting with dairy first. Further information about managing allergic proctocolitis can be found at www.infantproctocolitis.org.

IgE-mediated reactions to food proteins in breastmilk are much less common. These infants may develop eczema, wheezing, hives, blow out stools, vomiting, failure-to-thrive or anaphylaxis. If such allergic symptoms are present, the infant should be evaluated by an allergist. In the meantime, mom could avoid foods in her diet that family members are known to be allergic to, since food allergies can be genetic.

Infant Illness Or Surgery

Infants should continue to breastfeed when ill, unless unable to take anything by mouth. Infants who are vomiting are also encouraged to continue breastfeeding ad lib. Mother may need to pump to maintain her supply if her infant is unable or unwilling to breastfeed effectively. Infants needing general anesthesia should be allowed to breastfeed up until 4 hours prior to the procedure. A helpful guideline is the Academy of Breastfeeding Medicine's protocol entitled 'Preprocedural Fasting for the Breastfed Infant', http://www.bfmed.org/Resources/Protocols.aspx

Breast Refusal

This is very distressing for mothers, and often requires referral to a lactation specialist.

If infant has never latched, spending as much time as possible skin-to-skin with an infant of any age can help trigger the innate reflexes to find a breast and latch on. Breastfeeding is a very instinctual behavior, such that infants don't lose the ability to latch during the first year or so. Some infants don't latch-on and nurse for the first time until 4-6 months of age.

If an infant had been nursing, and stopped, it is important to identify WHY the infant is refusing to latch. Possible reasons include fear of a high milk supply and fast flow, frustration about a low milk supply and the resulting slow flow, inability to remove milk well, or simply a preference for the fast and even flow of bottles. A lactation specialist can help address each of these issues.

If an infant has been breastfeeding successfully for months and suddenly refuses the breast, the infant is likely on a 'nursing strike'. This can happen for many reasons, but most commonly can be a response to mother's return to work. The infant may decide that he likes bottles better, or he may be frustrated with mom's drop in milk supply. Sometimes a nursing strike may result from infant illness, teething, a fright such as mom's reaction from an infant bite to the nipple, or from the taste of a cream used on the nipples. One strategy is to feed most of the feeding with a bottle, and then offer a breast, when the infant is relaxed and no longer hungry. 'Dream feeding' is also a strategy. This involves offering the breast just as the infant is falling asleep or waking up, calling upon the infant's innate nursing instinct.

Reasons for refusing only one breast may be related to infant discomfort. These problems can include torticollis, a broken clavicle or a subdural hematoma in a newborn. Infants may also show preference of one breast because of significant differences in milk production between breasts. Younger infants may refuse a faster-flowing breast, and older infants often refuse the slower flowing one. A pump may be needed to try and even out production, unless mom is happy to let the slower/rejected side dry up completely. The breasts do work independently, and this is possible, but some mothers do not like to appear "lop-sided".

Nipple Shield Use

Nipple shields are covers made of pliable silicone that fit over the nipple/areolar complex. They are firmer than the breast and allow the breast to feel more like the bottle when the infant latches on. The silicone provides a firm stimulus to the infant's palate, which wakes the infant and can encourage the infant to stay latched on and suck.

However, there are significant problems with the nipple shield:

- Once moms introduce a nipple shield, it can be very difficult for the infant to nurse without it.
- There might be a decreased transfer of milk from the breast to the infant, especially when mom's milk supply is low or marginal. This might be due to the infant's inability to both accommodate the shield in his mouth, and reach mother's glandular tissue behind the areola.
- The nipple shield might blunt mom's nipple from feeling the infant nursing at the breast.

This decrease in nipple sensation might theoretically reduce mom's prolactin level.

- The nipple shield can cause a decrease in milk supply. Mothers ought to be instructed to pump after nursing with a nipple shield to preserve her milk supply, unless she has difficulty with an oversupply.

- Some mothers who have sore nipples experience more pain when using a nipple shield, because the infant is unable to latch deeply while using the shield. Superficial latching while using the shield causes the nipple to become compressed within the layers of the nipple shield.

- For all of the above reasons, nipple shield use should be supervised by lactation specialists who have evaluated both mom and infant and have given informed consent to mom about the risk of using a nipple shield.

Bottle Refusal

Offering the newborn a bottle once breastfeeding is well established, by 3-4 weeks of age, helps to decrease the risk of bottle refusal. This is a very distressing problem for families and daycare providers. Sometimes infants will accept cup feeding, or they will take a bottle when very relaxed. Some infants refuse to take any expressed breastmilk, and will wait until reunited with the mother to feed. These infants will often reverse-cycle nurse, with frequent night-time feedings. For a handout on tips for bottle refusal, please see https://themilkmob.org/

and choose "Breastfeeding Handouts" from the "Learn" menu.

Infant Tongue-Tie

Ankyloglossia can cause nipple soreness and damage, starting as early as the first day postpartum. Please see Pg. 37 for more details on anterior vs posterior tongue-ties.

If a tongue-tie is not clipped in the first few weeks, the mother and infant should be monitored closely over the course of the next 6 months, to ensure proper infant growth and maintenance of maternal milk supply. In the first few months postpartum, mother's milk supply is somewhat high, such that the infant may not need to work very hard to draw sufficient milk. As mother's baseline prolactin declines over time, milk removal depends more on the infant's deep latch and ability to express milk by compressing and massaging the breast tissue behind the areola. If an infant with a tongue-tie is not able to latch deeply, there may be an insidious drop in maternal milk supply and infant weight over time, first noticeable at 2-4 months postpartum. This may be an indication for clipping the tongue-tie, even if mother does not experience nipple pain. A helpful guideline is the Academy of Breastfeeding Medicine's Protocol entitled 'Guidelines for the evaluation and management of neonatal ankyloglossia and its complications in the breastfeeding dyad'. http://www.bfmed.org/Resources/Protocols.aspx

Special-Needs Infants

Down Syndrome (Trisomy 21)

Infants with Down syndrome can have difficulty with effective milk removal due to low muscle tone. Infants with Down syndrome are often poor feeders and slow gainers regardless of how they are fed. Supporting both of the infant's cheeks with mother's thumb and first finger while supporting the breast with the palm and remaining fingers can help increase intra-oral pressure and deepen the latch. Because of oral abnormalities, malocclusion, and neurocognitive impairment, breastfeeding is very important to optimize health and cognitive outcomes for this population.

Please see the Academy of Breastfeeding Medicine protocol 'Breastfeeding the Hypotonic Infant' http://www.bfmed.org/Resources/Protocols.aspx

Cleft Lip and Palate

Infants with a cleft palate usually have difficulty forming a sufficient seal to complete all feeding from the breast. However, each infant should be evaluated on an individual basis. Special bottles are usually needed to sustain adequate weight gain for this population. Breastmilk is very important for infants with a cleft palate, in order to minimize the risk of middle ear infections, and to optimize healing after surgical repair of the palate.

Feeding at the breast is more successful in infants with a cleft lip only as long as attention is paid to creating a seal at the site of the defect. It may help to hand express before a feeding if the breast is very firm. This helps the breast conform to the defect, so infant can create suction to express milk from the breast. Many surgeons will allow the infant to breastfeed immediately after surgical repair.

More information is available in the Academy of Breastfeeding Medicine Protocol 'Guidelines for Breastfeeding Infants with Cleft Lip, Cleft Palate, or Cleft Lip and Palate, Revised 2013' http://www.bfmed.org/Resources/Protocols.aspx

Congenital Heart Disease

Infants with cardiac problems often need to have milk volume and calories closely monitored. They benefit from short frequent feeds to prevent fatigue. As with premature infants, the work of breastfeeding is less than that of bottle feeding. Studies have shown an improved oxygen saturation with breastfeeding the infant with cardiac problems. To limit fluid intake while boosting calories, mom can set aside the milk from the first five minutes of a pumping session, allowing the milk to separate and the cream to rise to the top. That cream can be added to another bottle of milk and the bottle swirled gently to mix.

Metabolic Disorders

Sometimes infants with metabolic disorders, such as MCADD (medium chain acyl-CoA dehydrogenase deficiency), are able to breastfeed. Weights need to be monitored closely for appropriate growth.

Type 1 galactosemia is a contraindication to breastfeeding and breastmilk. The Duarte variant of galactosemia may be compatible with partial breastfeeding if there is enough enzyme present. Consultation with a pediatric metabolic specialist is important for any infant with a metabolic disorder.

Complementary Feeding

Infants are ready for solids, or complementary feeding, at 6 months of age.

Complementary foods ought to be high in iron, as infants beyond 6 months need additional sources of iron beyond breastmilk. Iron-rich foods include red meat, poultry, fish, legumes, spinach, sweet potatoes, prunes, and iron-fortified cereals.

There is no other recommendation on what foods to introduce first. Complementary feedings should reflect the foods that are typically eaten by the family, assuming healthy choices. A wide variety of fruits, vegetables, grains, and proteins will ensure adequate intake of nutrients. The World Health Organization recommends 2-3 meals a day for infants 6-8 months of age, and 3-4 meals a day for infants 9-23 months of age, with 1-2 additional snacks as required.

Breastfeeding should continue frequently and on-demand during complementary feeding, until at least 2 years of age or beyond. For more details on complementary feeding, please see the World Health Organization Global Strategy for Infant and Young Feeding:
http://who.int/nutrition/topics/global_strategy_iycf/en/

Exclusive Pumping

There are many reasons why a mother exclusively pumps her milk and does not nurse. Common reasons include pain with nursing, and infant inability or refusal to nurse. Women with a history of sexual abuse may be uncomfortable putting the infant to the breast. Women need to learn how to use their pump properly to avoid pump trauma and to ensure good milk drainage.

Risks of exclusively pumping include plugged ducts due to uneven or insufficient breast drainage, nipple pain and trauma, insufficient milk supply, and excessive milk supply.

When babies breastfeed, they take the amount of milk that they need. If the mother generates more milk than a nursing infant needs, the lack of complete breast emptying feeds back to the milk-producing cells in order to bring the supply down. Many mothers who are exclusive pumpers drive their supplies up too high, because they tend to pump to complete emptying, which is a strong physiologic message to the cells to make more milk.

Every mother who is an exclusive pumper ought to receive counseling on proper breast shield size, ideal pump pressure settings, and recommendations on duration and frequency of pumping, depending on her milk supply and her capabilities.

Pump Technology

Choosing a breast pump can be a confusing task. Since approximately 2012, many insurance companies in the USA have been mandated to supply breast pumps, and many mothers do not have a choice of breast pumps unless one is purchased in addition to what her insurance supplies. Many WIC agencies (Special Supplemental Nutrition Program for Women, Infants and Children) also supply pumps to breastfeeding mothers.

Breast pumps can be single sided and manually operated (hand pumps). Most women choose pumps that express both breasts at the same time (double-electric) using electricity, disposable batteries, or a rechargeable battery. Some pumps only allow mothers to have control over the degree of suction. Other pumps also allow mothers to control the speed of the suction cycles. Many pumps have a 'stimulation phase', which is a fast, low-suction cycle. This is designed to encourage a milk ejection reflex. Once the milk begins flowing, it is typically recommended that the mother switch the setting to the 'expression phase', which has a slower cycle and increased suction for more efficient and complete emptying.

'Hospital grade' pumps are expensive multiuser pumps with good quality motors. The FDA does not have a definition for 'hospital grade'. These pumps have a closed system, meaning that milk cannot flow from the pump collection kit into the pump itself, preventing contamination from one user to another. There are several newer pumps on the market that are closed systems with excellent motors at a reasonable price, making the cost of renting a hospital grade pump often unnecessary, since the more expensive rental pumps have not been shown to be more effective than these newer higher quality pumps on the market. An exception may be for mothers of premature infants, since some of the newer hospital grade pumps have patented cycle patterns for mothers with premature infants. There is not a great deal of research on the true efficacy of these patented cycles.

Every mother needs to learn how to use her breast pump properly, to prevent nipple trauma and loss of milk supply due to insufficient drainage. This involves making sure that the breast shield, which is the flange into which the breast is placed, is properly fitted. Most breast pumps offer different breast shield sizes, and some pumps have soft flexible shields that are one-size-fits-all.

The instructions on how long to pump at what suction level is also very individual, depending on the reason for pumping and maternal physiologic factors such as speed of letdown and milk supply. It is recommended that mothers use the highest suction strength that is still comfortable. Just as we encourage every new mother to be observed while nursing to ensure proper latch and good milk transfer, a mother who is relying heavily on pumping for milk expression would benefit from being observed while pumping to ensure safe and effective pump use.

Milk Storage

Mothers should wash their hands and use clean pump parts before pumping for milk storage. Milk that has less bacterial contamination at the time of milk expression will have higher protein levels and less bacterial growth when left at room temperature fresh or after thawing.

The breasts do not need to be cleansed before milk expression.

BPA-free hard plastic or glass containers are ideal for milk storage in the freezer. If plastic bags are used, they should be sturdy and made for milk storage. Double-bagging milk can reduce the risk of bag punctures.

Expressed breastmilk will normally separate, with cream on the top. The milk can be gently swirled to distribute the fat in the milk before infant feeding.

Location of Storage	Temp	Maximum Duration of Storage
Room Temperature	~60-85° F (15-30°C)	3-4 hour optimal, up to 6-8 hours in very clean conditions and cooler room temperatures
Refrigerator	~39°F (4°C)	72 hours optimal
Freezer	<0°F (-17°C)	6 months optimal, 12 months acceptable

Very little research has been done on the safety of milk storage at 55°C, which is the estimated temperature in a cooler pack. Given that freshly expressed breastmilk appears safe for up to 6-8 hours at room temperature, storage in a cooler bag should be fine for 8 hours.

Thawing frozen milk is best done slowly, such as in the refrigerator overnight. Thawing in warm water can reduce the fat content, so using lukewarm water rather than hot water is safest, to avoid excessive melting of the milk fat, which causes adherence to the wall of the containers.

Once milk is thawed in the refrigerator, it is best to use it within 1-2 days.

Reheating thawed breastmilk is also best accomplished with low heat such as a lukewarm water bath.

Breastmilk should never be microwaved. Microwaving can cause hot spots in milk, and can denature the bioactive proteins, reducing the immunological properties in breastmilk.

Unfinished bottle feedings should be discarded if not used within an hour or two. Re-refrigeration of left-over thawed milk is not currently recommended.

Returning to Work or School

Mothers are encouraged to take as much time off as possible for maternity leave, in order to recover from delivery and to establish a strong milk supply. Tips for mothers returning to work include:

- The mother is encouraged to contact her employer regarding her lactation needs, such as a pumping schedule, lactation room and possibly transitioning back to work part-time.

- Find a supportive daycare that is comfortable with breastmilk storage, and who will support her with her goals of breastfeeding her child.

- Begin storing an extra 1-2 ounces of breastmilk a day approximately 1 month before returning to work. Store in 2-4 ounce increments.

- Introduce a bottle to the infant before returning to work, or by 4 weeks of age to decrease chance of bottle refusal.

- Plan her pumping schedule before returning to work. Plan to pump approximately every 3 hours when the infant is under 6 months. She may be able to pump less often such as every 4 hours after 6 months, once the infant is taking solids.

- Have access to a good quality double electric breast pump that allows for efficient breast drainage in 10-15 minutes.

Maternal Medications

Very few medications are contraindicated during lactation. On average, a very small percent of the maternal dose reaches the infant, and is usually not clinically significant. Drug transfer depends on oral bioavailability, molecular weight, protein binding, and lipid solubility. If a drug is not absorbed orally, it is obviously not a concern for the infant. Some drug molecules are too large, or too protein-bound to pass into the milk compartment. Most drugs in maternal serum pass into the milk by equilibration, meaning that a high concentration in the serum leads to a high concentration in the milk. As the serum level drops, most drugs pass back from the milk into the serum.

The age and medical condition of the child, as well as the frequency of nursing, are also considerations in the decisions regarding the safety of any medication. Medications that are FDA-approved for use in infants should pose little concern. If a specific drug is not a good choice, often there is a related drug (with a shorter half-life for instance) that would be a better alternative. In rare situations, it is appropriate to "pump and dump" milk for the course of treatment and resume breastfeeding afterwards. Some radiopharmaceuticals fall into this category.

It is also important to consider a medication's effect on mother's milk production. Many medications decrease the milk supply, such as hormonal contraceptives, strong antihistamines, high dose steroids, and pseudoephedrine.

Psychiatric medications are commonly prescribed for lactating women, and should be accompanied by counseling when indicated. Any medication that increases dopamine will decrease the prolactin level, and thus the milk supply. The Academy of Breastfeeding Medicine has a helpful protocol entitled 'Use of Antidepressants in Breastfeeding Mothers'
http://www.bfmed.org/Resources/Protocols.aspx

Clinicians need to know where to find the latest information on medications during lactation:

- The LACTMED database at the National Library of Medicine's toxnet website https://toxnet.nlm.nih.gov/newtoxnet/lactmed.htm. This is a free database, accessible to anyone, and frequently updated
- 'Medications and Mother's Milk' handbook by Thomas Hale PhD, RPh
- The Infant Risk Center www.infantrisk.com
- The Organization of Teratology Information Specialists - Mothertobaby.org

Herbal Medications

As medicinal use of herbs becomes more common, it is helpful to have a resource when questions from lactating mothers arise. In general, it is safest to avoid herbs while lactating, if possible, as they are not well-regulated in the US. Helpful resources include: www.herbmed.org , http://nccam.nih.gov, www.naturaldatabase.com, and https://toxnet.nlm.nih.gov/newtoxnet/lactmed.htm

Recreational Substances

Drugs of abuse are generally contraindicated in nursing mothers. One possible exception may be occasional marijuana use. Because we know the active components of marijuana are excreted in breastmilk and concentrate in the developing brain of infants, marijuana use in lactation should definitely be discouraged. Exposure to the smoke itself should also be avoided. But the risk of completely weaning because of occasional marijuana use may be greater than the risk of not breastfeeding. Research on this topic is a work in progress. Latest information is available at Lactmed, the Infant Risk Center, and Mothertobaby.org, as listed above.

Alcohol

Alcohol passes freely into and out of the milk, so a mother's blood alcohol level is essentially equal to her milk alcohol level at any moment in time. As she metabolizes the ingested alcohol, it passes back out of the milk compartment into the blood. Alcohol intake also decreases the amount of breastmilk an infant removes from the breast. Chronic alcohol use decreases milk supply as well as increases the risk of adverse cognitive effects for the infant.

Reasonable advice would be no more than 2 drinks per day, and not daily, with each drink over 2 hours. It is also helpful to eat food while drinking, to decrease the rate of absorption. Exposure to the infant can be further minimized by waiting at least 2 hours after the last drink to breastfeed. For special occasions where more 2 drinks are consumed in an evening, milk can be expressed and discarded to help maintain supply while decreasing infant exposure. One "serving" of alcohol = 12 oz beer, 5 oz wine, or 1.5 oz 80-proof spirits.

<u>Smoking</u>

Exposure should be minimized, and nicotine patches to aid in smoking cessation are preferable to cigarettes. Smoking decreases milk supply, and increases the infant's risk of SIDS. Smoking is also an independent risk factor for early breastfeeding cessation.

Multiples

Mothers with multiple infants are often able to completely nurse their infants without supplementation. It is reasonable to encourage mothers with multiples to hand express colostrum after feedings in the first few days. This sends a strong signal to the breasts to maximize milk production. It is often easier for mother and newborns to nurse one at a time in the early days. As the mother becomes more comfortable with positioning and latching her newborns, she can work on her tandem nursing skills, meaning nursing two infants at the same time. Special pillows made to support twins help immensely with positioning and maternal comfort. Mother should be encouraged to arrange for extra help at home, as she will be working full time to breastfeed and/or express milk for her infants.

Induced and Re-Lactation

Re-lactation means to start breastfeeding again sometime after weaning. This is most common in situations where mom has weaned or lost her supply due to illness or other circumstances and then decides that she would like to start nursing again and needs help re-establishing her milk supply.

Many mothers who had a healthy milk supply are able to reestablish lactation. These mothers need comprehensive evaluation by a lactation specialist, to establish a plan for restoring their supply.

Induced lactation is the process of bringing on lactation without going through pregnancy and birth. Adoption and surrogacy are the most common reasons to pursue this. Induced lactation is most successful in moms who have been pregnant in the past, or who have lactated/breastfed in the past. The process often can involve:

- Hormone preparation, often with birth control pills, to simulate pregnancy.
- Galactogogues, either herbal or prescription, to increase the prolactin level.
- Frequent pumping for several weeks after stopping the birth control pill, before the infant arrives, to stimulate milk production.

An informational website on adoptive nursing is http://www.breastfeedingwithoutbirthing.com/

Tandem Nursing

Some mothers continue to nurse their older child through their pregnancy and after the birth of their new infant. If the older nursling is under one year while mother is pregnant, he must have his weight closely monitored and may need supplementation, as many mothers experience a significant decrease in their milk supply during the pregnancy. As the due date approaches, the milk will change to meet the new infant's needs and after birth the supply will adjust according to the needs of both nurslings. The mother should be advised to allow her infant to feed first in the early days, to be sure the newborn's needs are prioritized. Once mature milk production is reestablished, there should be plenty for both nurslings.

Weaning

Technically, weaning begins the moment complementary foods (or formula) are offered to an infant. Too often, weaning occurs earlier than desired due to misinformation, or the infant refuses the breast because the flow is too slow. There is no maximum time limit on breastfeeding. All major health organizations recommend that infants nurse until at least one year of age and many recommend nursing until at least two years of age. Breastmilk has important nutritional and immunologic value for the entire duration of breastfeeding. Many of the "benefits" are dose responsive, meaning the longer the child breastfeeds, the healthier he has the potential to be. And as the daily volume of milk decreases, many of the protective factors actually increase in concentration.

Weaning is the process of gradually reducing the frequency of breastfeeding, so that the infant is gradually taking less breastmilk in her diet.

If possible, weaning more gradually is preferred. This can be accomplished by slowly eliminating feedings or pumping sessions, while leaving milk in the breasts to slow production. If a mom is exclusively pumping, she could gradually decrease the amount removed at each pumping session. With a toddler, the "don't offer, don't refuse" method can be used, with the goal of eliminating one daily feed per week. Distracting the toddler with another activity, or leaving the house can be helpful. Usually the last feeding at night and the first in the morning are the nursing sessions toddlers hold onto the longest.

Babies are healthiest when they can continue to be breastfed until at least one year of age or longer, but sometimes mothers need or decide to wean earlier for many different reasons.

Mothers do not need to fully wean their infants from the breast when they decrease the frequency of breastfeeding. A mother can decide to nurse her infant less often, such as three to four times a day, rather than eight times a day, and still continue to nurse the infant for a year or longer. She will have less milk if she nurses less often, and will need to supplement with formula. However, she will continue to lactate until she completely stops nursing and/or expressing her milk.

Weaning should be a personal decision by the mother, and not a decision made by other family members. A mother should not feel ashamed, cajoled or threatened into weaning her infant. Breastfeeding is the greatest first gift a mother can give to her infant. Breastfeeding allows for optimal infant and maternal health. Comments made to mothers about weaning are most often based on myth, cultural bias and are not respectful to the mother and infant.

Infant-Led Weaning

Infant-led weaning means that the mother allows the infant or toddler to take the lead on when weaning happens. This may happen at 8-10 months of age, as the infant becomes more mobile and busy. The infant may be more interested in exploring her environment and eating at the table rather than in mom's lap. Infant-led weaning more commonly occurs after 1 year of age. A mother who takes weaning cues from her toddler might allow the child to nurse whenever he wants to, and as he loses interest, he will nurse less over time.

Mother-Led Weaning

This method involves the mother initiating the weaning. The mother drops a nursing session and instead feeds the infant stored breastmilk, donor milk, or formula. Her body will adjust to skipping that feeding session in a few days. At that point, she can drop another nursing session at an opposite time of the day, and again allow her body to adjust before continuing to drop additional nursing sessions. Once she drops her last nursing session, she may need to express her milk to provide comfort for a day or two. It will often take at least two weeks for a mother to fully wean from nursing.

If the mother prefers to stop nursing immediately, she can wean via pumping. She would pump to comfort at regular intervals, such as every four hours. The breasts should not be fully emptied. Once she is comfortable with every four hours, she should decrease to every six hours, then eventually every eight hours, then ten hours, etc. The speed of weaning depends on how her breasts adjust. Her breasts should be comfortable without excessive engorgement before increasing the intervals between pumping.

Abrupt Weaning

Occasionally women need to wean abruptly due to a new maternal illness such as cancer, or for infant death. If her milk supply is well established, it is best for her to be treated with a medication to reduce her milk supply, such as pseudoephedrine 30mg 2-3 times a day as tolerated, or cabergoline 0.25mg every 3 days as needed. A well fitting bra and ice packs will also help discomfort.

Mothers who have suffered infant death might find milk donation very meaningful and comforting as a means of coping with their loss. Many milk banks associated with the Human Milk Banking Association of North America (hmbana.org) have bereavement support programs for these mothers.

Keeping the Breasts Comfortable During Weaning

When the breasts feel uncomfortably full, mom should either manually express or pump just to comfort. Leaving the breasts somewhat full tells the breasts that milk is no longer needed. The body then decides to make less milk.

Cold compresses can help to reduce engorgement and a hot shower can help to release extra milk when feeling too full. Some medications can reduce the milk supply, namely decongestants such as pseudoephedrine and the birth control pill with estrogen.

Natural substances can also reduce the supply. Peppermint is one option, such as strong lozenges or peppermint tea. The herb sage also can reduce the supply. Sage can be purchased as an extract, tea, or as a fresh or dried herb which can be added to food.

Weaning the Toddler Who Loves to Nurse

Weaning a toddler who loves to nurse can be one of the greatest breastfeeding challenges for a mom. Children who breastfeed into toddlerhood often nurse for comfort, security, and relaxation, as well as for nutrition. Strategies include:

- If the toddler is still nursing whenever he chooses, first try a breastfeeding schedule so that the child is only nursing at times that are ideal for mom, such as upon awakening, before and after naps, and at bedtime. Sometimes this is liberating for a mother, so that she feels sufficiently in control of breastfeeding.

- Once the toddler is on a nursing schedule, start dropping nursing sessions.

- Distract the toddler with toys, books, or a special treat when the toddler wants to nurse.

- Some toddlers adjust best if mom is not around at the time of a dropped feeding.

- Changing the toddler's routine may also help, such as having another adult such as dad putting the child to bed rather than mom.

Donor Human Milk

There are several means for families to donate and receive donor milk.

Banked, Pasteurized Donor Human Milk

Most of the milk banks in the USA are non-profit and are associated with the Human Milk Banking Association of North America (HMBANA). Only a few milk banks are for-profit. Mothers who are interested in donating their extra breastmilk are screened via interview and blood testing for infectious diseases, medications, and life style habits, just as individuals who donate blood. HMBANA milk banks request letters of approval from the infant's and mother's physician. The HMBANA milk banks pool, pasteurize and refreeze the donated milk. Most of the milk is sold and shipped to hospital neonatal intensive care units, and a sizeable amount is sold for outpatient use.

Unpasteurized Donor Breastmilk

Families who are interested in obtaining donor breastmilk for their outpatient infants need guidance on how to do this safely. Due to the high cost, purchasing pasteurized donor human milk from a milk bank is usually beyond the financial means for most families. Advising a family to refuse breastmilk from a donor other than a breastmilk bank increases the risk that the family may accept donor milk from unsafe sources. In these situations, it is best to advise families that it is safest to accept milk from donors who they know and trust, such as sisters, other relatives, or close friends. Families receiving unpasteurized, unscreened donor milk should ask the donor about medications, use of alcohol, tobacco, and illicit drugs, and consider screening for infectious illnesses, primarily HIV and HTLV 1 and 2. Families should never pay for donor milk from sources other than a HMBANA milk bank. Sellers of breastmilk have a conflict of interest, increasing the risk of watering down or adding animal milk to the breastmilk. Families should not seek or obtain breastmilk via the internet or from someone who the family does not know.

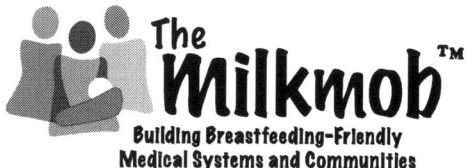

The **Milk Mob**

Building Breastfeeding-Friendly Medical Systems and Communities

The Milk Mob is a 501(c)3 nonprofit membership organization whose mission is to optimize the promotion and support of breastfeeding for families in the outpatient sector. The Milk Mob is dedicated to building Breastfeeding Friendly Medical Systems and Communities, through:

- Education of medical staff, providers, and other outpatient community breastfeeding supporters,

- Guidance in the development and sustainment of breastfeeding support networks within medical systems,

- Collaboration of breastfeeding support between hospitals, outpatient medical systems and community institutions for collective impact,

- Provision of educational resources for breastfeeding educators, such as sharing of educational materials, creation of audiovisual media, and tools for community supporters that promote consistent, evidence-based support of breastfeeding dyads.

Learn more at themilkmob.org

Bibliography

Would you really want the bibliography for this book in your pocket? We wouldn't, so we put it online at our website. You can view it, along with other Little-Green-Book-related info at:

 https://themilkmob.org/lgb/

Breastfeeding Resources

Yep! Also too big for this book.
For a comprehensive list of reliable sources for further breastfeeding education, visit our reference page at:

https://themilkmob.org/milk-mob-breastfeeding-education-handouts/basic-breastfeeding-information/

The Milk Mob Online Training for Physicians and other Providers

 https://themilkmob.org/providers-course/

Academy of Breastfeeding Medicine Protocols

http://www.bfmed.org/Resources/Protocols.aspx

Breastfeeding Medicine Podcast

 https://themilkmob.org/podcasts/

The Authors

Anne Eglash MD, IBCLC, FABM, is a clinical professor with the University of Wisconsin School of Medicine and Public Health, in the Department of Family and Community Medicine. In addition to practicing family medicine, she has been a board certified lactation consultant since 1994.

Dr. Eglash is a cofounder of the Academy of Breastfeeding Medicine, the Medical Director and cofounder of the Mothers' Milk Bank of the Western Great Lakes, and the Medical Director of the University of Wisconsin Lactation Services. She has published many peer- reviewed articles on breastfeeding medicine.

She co-hosts and produces a breastfeeding medicine podcast series, called The Breastfeeding Medicine Podcast, available free on i-tunes and The Milk Mob website.

Dr. Eglash is founder and president of The Milk Mob, a nonprofit organization dedicated to the creation of breastfeeding-friendly medical systems and communities.

Kathy Leeper, MD, IBCLC, FABM first worked as a general pediatrician, then helped develop a nonprofit breastfeeding center in Lincoln, Nebraska called MilkWorks, which opened in 2001. She served as its Medical Director, practicing breastfeeding medicine exclusively until 2014. After moving to Kansas City, KS in 2014, she joined the Milk Mob to serve on the board of directors, as a trainer and to help with the development of new educational material.

She currently serves on the Board of Directors of the Academy of Breastfeeding Medicine.

Gail S. Hertz, MD, IBCLC, FABM is a pediatrician. She attended Penn State College of Medicine, graduating in 1997 and did her residency at Penn State Children's Hospital in Hershey, PA. She has been an Internationally Board Certified Lactation Consultant since 1998.

She was inspired to write the original Little Green Book when she was pumping milk for her daughter during her first year of medical school.

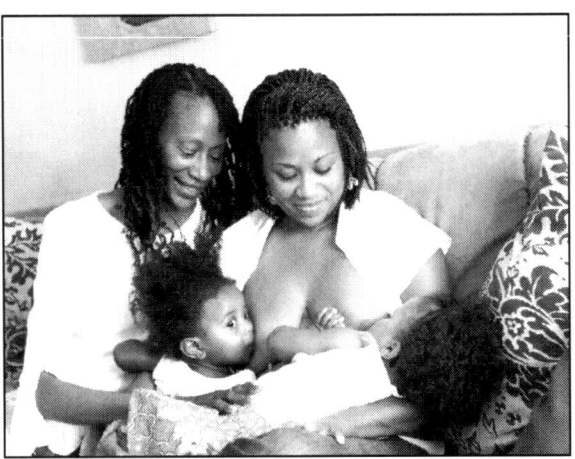

Image Courtesy United States Breastfeeding Committee

Index

A

B

C

D

E

F

O

Obesity, morbid 10, 20, 63
Opioids 18
Oxytocin 17, 65

P

Pacifiers 21, 27
Pain, breast, nipple 35, 51, 58, 59
Phenylketonuria 13
Physiology 15
Placenta 15, 63, 64, 70
Plugged ducts 55, 59, 60, 69, 85
Polycystic ovarian syndrome 20
Positioning to breastfeed 24, 35
Postpartum depression 73
Prematurity 40
Prenatal counseling 18
Proctocolitis 77
Progesterone 16, 64, 70
Prolactin 16, 46, 67, 69, 70, 80, 81, 91, 95
Pseudoephedrine 69, 91

R

Re-lactation 94
Return to work 89
Reverse pressure softening 50
Risks of formula feeding 10
Rooming-In 21, 25

S

T

V

W